D0292444

HUMANITARIAN NEGOTIATIONS REVEALED

CLAIRE MAGONE, MICHAEL NEUMAN,
FABRICE WEISSMAN

(*Editors*)

Humanitarian Negotiations Revealed

The MSF Experience

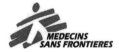

Médecins Sans Frontières

HURST & COMPANY, LONDON

First published in the United Kingdom in 2011 by
C. Hurst & Co. (Publishers) Ltd.,
41 Great Russell Street, London, WC1B 3PL
© Médecins Sans Frontières, 2011
All rights reserved.
Printed in India by Imprint Digital

The right of Mědecins Sans Frontières to be identified as the
authors of this publication is asserted by it in accordance with
the Copyright, Designs and Patents Act, 1988.

A Cataloguing-in-Publication data record for this book
is available from the British Library.

ISBN: 978-1-84904-163-8 paperback
      978-1-84904-162-1 hardback

This book is printed using paper from registered sustainable
and managed sources.

www.hurstpub.co.uk

ALSO FROM MEDECINS SANS FRONTIERES

François Jean (ed.), *Populations in Danger* (London: John Libbey, 1992).

François Jean (ed.), *Life, Death and Aid: The Médecins Sans Frontières Report on World Crisis Intervention* (London: Routledge, 1993).

François Jean (ed.), *Populations in Danger 1995: A Médecins Sans Frontières Report* (Paris & London: 1995).

Julia Groenwald (ed.), *World in Crisis. The Politics of Survival at the End of the Twentieth Century* (London: Routledge, 1996).

Fabrice Weissman (ed.), *In the Shadow of Just Wars. Violence, Politics and Humanitarian Action* (London: Hurst &Co., 2004).

Xavier Crombé and Jean-Hervé Jézéquel (eds), *A Not So Natural Disaster: Niger 2005* (London: Hurst & Co., 2009).

CONTENTS

CONTENTS

PART II: HISTORY

ABOUT THE CONTRIBUTORS

Marie-Pierre Allié, a medical doctor, is the president of the French section of Médecins Sans Frontières.

Caroline Abu-Sada is the coordinator of the Research Unit of the Swiss section of Médecins Sans Frontières.

Laurence Binet is a director of studies at the Centre de réflexion sur l'action et les savoirs humanitaires, Fondation Médecins Sans Frontières.

Jean-Hervé Bradol, a medical doctor, is a director of studies at the Centre de réflexion sur l'action et les savoirs humanitaires, Fondation Médecins Sans Frontières. He is a former president of the French section of Médecins Sans Frontières (2000–2008).

Rony Brauman, a medical doctor, is a director of studies at the Centre de réflexion sur l'action et les savoirs humanitaires, Fondation Médecins Sans Frontières. He is a former president of the French section of Médecins Sans Frontières (1982–1994).

Xavier Crombé is a lecturer at Sciences Po in Paris. He is a former head of mission for Médecins Sans Frontières in Afghanistan (2002–2003) and a former director of studies at the Centre de réflexion sur l'action et les savoirs humanitaires, Fondation Médecins Sans Frontières (2005–2008).

Stéphane Doyon is the nutrition team leader at the Campaign for Access to Essential Medicines of Médecins Sans Frontières.

Michiel Hofman is a former head of mission for Médecins Sans Frontières in Afghanistan (2009–2011).

ABOUT THE CONTRIBUTORS

Michel-Olivier Lacharité is a programme manager for Médecins Sans Frontières.

Benoît Leduc is a former programme manager for Médecins Sans Frontières (2007–2010).

Marc Le Pape is a sociologist and a former member of the Board of the French section of Médecins Sans Frontières (1998–2008).

Claire Magone is a director of studies at the Centre de réflexion sur l'action et les savoirs humanitaires, Fondation Médecins Sans Frontières.

Michaël Neuman is a director of studies at the Centre de réflexion sur l'action et les savoirs humanitaires, Fondation Médecins Sans Frontières.

David Rieff is an independent journalist, author of *A Bed for the Night. Humanitarianism in Crisis* (New York: Simon & Schuster, 2003).

Fiona Terry is an independent researcher and a former director of studies at the Centre de réflexion sur l'action et les savoirs humanitaires, Fondation Médecins Sans Frontières.

Claudine Vidal is a sociologist, Groupe de sociologie politique et morale, École des hautes études en sciences sociales.

Fabrice Weissman is a director of studies at the Centre de réflexion sur l'action et les savoirs humanitaires, Fondation Médecins Sans Frontières.

Jonathan Whittall is a humanitarian adviser at Médecins Sans Frontières—South Africa.

LIST OF MAPS

ABBREVIATIONS

EU	European Union
ICRC	International Committee of the Red Cross
IMF	International Monetary Fund
MSF	Médecins Sans Frontières
NGO	Non-Governmental Organisation
OCHA	Office for the Coordination of Humanitarian Affairs
UN	United Nations
UNICEF	United Nations Children's Fund
UNHCR	United Nations High Commissioner for Refugees (or HCR: High Commissioner for Refugees)
WFP	World Food Programme
WHO	World Health Organization

ACKNOWLEDGMENTS

This book is a collective effort. Marc Le Pape and Claudine Vidal, as well as all our colleagues and interns at the Centre de réflexion sur l'action et les savoirs humanitaires (CRASH/Fondation MSF), have all made invaluable contributions to this project. Caroline Serraf organised the translations, which were proofread and edited with painstaking care by Ros Smith-Thomas. This book would not have been possible without the enthusiastic collaboration of the Médecins Sans Frontières coordinators in the field and at headquarters.

All are warmly thanked.

Paris, July 2011   C. M., M. N., F. W.

INTRODUCTION

ACTING AT ANY PRICE?

Marie-Pierre Allié
President of the French section of Médecins Sans Frontières

Between 2004 and 2008, nine members of Médecins Sans Frontières were killed in the course of their missions in Afghanistan, Central African Republic and Somalia. In 2008 and 2009, several MSF sections[1] had to leave Niger and the north of Sudan because the authorities had either suspended their activities or issued them with a deportation order. In 2009, under threat of expulsion from Sri Lanka, MSF signed a Memorandum of Understanding obliging it to remain silent—but still did not gain access to the combat zones. In Yemen, in January 2010, the organisation was forced to withdraw public statements deemed inaccurate and insulting by the government in order to keep its activities running.

Should we conclude from these events that the "humanitarian space" is shrinking, as many observers of the humanitarian scene have been claiming in recent years? NGOs, United Nations agencies and donors are unanimous in deploring a "growing tendency to close the door to humanitarians, preventing them from helping victims".[2] This would be in stark contrast with a so-called "golden age" when humanitarian actors supposedly occupied "a special position on the interna-

1

tional political chessboard, within a privileged space, untroubled by the geostrategic and political considerations of governments".[3] Since then, according to United Nations (UN) agencies, their space has been eroded by the "blurred distinctions between the roles of military and humanitarian organisations; political manipulation of humanitarian assistance [and the] perceived lack of independence of humanitarian actors from donors or from host governments".[4]

Since the end of the 1990s, MSF has also been vehemently denouncing the harm caused by the "blurring of lines", heightened with the revival of western military interventionism in the wake of 9/11, the development of international criminal justice and the integration of the aid system in the United Nations' political strategies. With their actions now equated with military, judicial and political forms of interventionism, NGOs such as MSF would be encountering increasing hostility in developing countries. They would be seemingly faced with a reaffirmation of sovereignty on the part of post-colonial states benefiting from the diplomatic and economic support of emerging powers.

This book does not set out to deny the consequences of belligerents using humanitarian rhetoric, or the fact that western aid organisations come up against specific difficulties in countries where international forces are deployed. But it does argue the impact of this environment on aid operations, if only on the grounds that the global volume of humanitarian assistance continues to grow. Between 1988 and 2008, the humanitarian aid budget increased ten-fold to reach 11.2 billion US dollars.[5] MSF's own operational spending rose from 260 million euros in 2001 to 634 million in 2010, most notably in Niger and Darfur (Sudan) where the organisation carried out two of the largest missions in its history. Furthermore, evoking a "golden age" in which aid actors were able to realise their ambitions unfettered is to underplay the very real difficulties encountered during the forced displacements in Ethiopia in the 1980s, for example, or, in the 1990s, the massacres in ex-Yugoslavia and the genocide in Rwanda.

Contrary to the "shrinking space" theory—which frees aid actors from any responsibility for conquering and defending their own sphere of activity—there are no legitimate perimeters to humanitarian action, valid at all times and in all situations, which become clearly visible once the mists of "military-humanitarian confusion" have lifted and humanitarians are protected from any political fallout. There is, however, a space for negotiation, power games and interest-seeking between aid actors and authorities. MSF's freedom of action is not rooted in a legal and moral "space of sovereignty" that simply needs to be proclaimed in order to be automatically acknowledged and respected. It is the product of repeated transactions with local and international political and military forces. Its scope depends largely on the organisation's ambitions, the diplomatic and political support it can rely on and the interest taken in its action by those in power.

This book follows on from the *Populations in Danger* series initiated by MSF under the direction of François Jean in 1992, and has been inspired by MSF's in-house debates on the evolution of its freedom of action. Eight years after the publication of *In the Shadow of Just Wars*,[6] it examines the precept that the political exploitation of aid is not a misuse of its vocation, but its principal condition of existence. If this is the case, how can MSF ensure that the negotiations it undertakes will result in an agreement it can live with? Because acknowledging that humanitarian aid is only possible when it coincides with the interests of the "powers that be" does not have to mean giving way to political forces. We are not looking to replace a school of thought that sees the humanitarian principles—independence, neutrality and impartiality—as a magic key to the humanitarian space with an attitude of ultra-pragmatism. Nor are we looking to transform adaptation to circumstance into an operational policy mantra.

But how can we judge whether a compromise is acceptable? We felt that this question should be examined in the light of MSF's concrete experience of negotiations by analysing the choices made by the organisation in specific situations of confrontation and collaboration. In doing so, the authors of this book have drawn on the association's archives, interviews with key protagonists and on their own experience, since most of them have worked with MSF in the field.

The chapters in the first part of the book describe specific negotiation situations. They contain a main case study and, in some cases, shorter pieces which help shed more light on the issue in question.

In each of these narratives, the authors highlight the shared and diverging interests of MSF, as a humanitarian medical organisation, and the political actors with whom it has to deal. What are these interests and what are the different motivations behind each party's action? For the organisation, they may involve providing impartial assistance to the direct victims of a conflict (Pakistan, Afghanistan, Palestinian Territories, Somalia, Sri Lanka, Ethiopia) and raising awareness of the violence of war in the hope of helping to attenuate it (Yemen, Ethiopia, Sri Lanka, Somalia, Palestinian Territories). They may also involve responding to the consequences of neglected public health problems (recurrent epidemics in Nigeria, malnutrition in India or AIDS in South Africa) or caring for populations who have been deliberately excluded from social and healthcare systems (migrants in France and ethnic minorities in Myanmar).

These ambitions may then come up against those of an army or a rebel movement using humanitarian aid as a means of gaining local or international legitimacy (Afghanistan, Pakistan, Palestinian Territories); those of foreign governments or international organisations seeking to isolate or strengthen a regime (Afghanistan, Somalia, Pakistan, Palestinian Territories) or those of armies or insurgents who make no distinction between combatants and non-combatants (Sri Lanka, Ethiopia, Yemen, Pakistan). MSF's objectives may also come up against those of authorities who are more concerned by the political consequences of an epidemic than by its consequences on health (Nigeria, South Africa); those of a government seeking the services of health workers to help it manage a system that excludes "undesirables" (Myanmar, France and Sri Lanka) or the ambitions of activist movements defending their vision of society (South Africa, India).

It is from such encounters of interests, sometimes opposing, sometimes convergent, that compromises are born. The justifications for these compromises need to be examined in context, but also within their broader environment. This is determined by the organisation's ambitions, the lessons it draws from its experiences in similar settings, and how it interacts with the other actors involved in managing armed conflict situations or health crises.

The chapters in the second part of the book describe the way MSF's choices have evolved in those categories of intervention that first led to the creation, in 1971, of an organisation made up "exclusively of doctors and members of the health sector" whose activity consists in assisting "victims of natural disasters, collective accidents and situations of belligerence".[7] MSF's objectives and practices in these contexts have been altered by the ideological confrontations it has taken part in during its existence, and by the way it sees its role within the organised international community—governments, interstate organisations and transnational NGOs. In their respective chapters, Fabrice Weissman, Jean-Hervé Bradol and Rony Brauman explain the way

INTRODUCTION

MSF has evolved over forty years of wars, public health policies and natural disasters. What does this journey through the contemporary narratives and long history of MSF tell us?

Everything is Open to Negotiation

As the interview with Benoît Leduc on MSF's project in Somalia demonstrates, "everything is open to negotiation". No parameter is fixed from the outset: the safety of personnel, the presence of expatriates, MSF's intervention priorities, the quality of the assistance provided, control over resources, etc. They are all the result of concessions, some justified by harsh realities—employing armed guards, for example—and others by their temporary nature, such as the remote management of programmes. Negotiation frameworks do not include universal markers indicating the line that must not be crossed; and MSF must therefore pay attention to the developing dynamic of each situation and to its own ability to revoke compromises that were only acceptable because they were temporary.

Judge for Ourselves

In negotiations concerning MSF's action, the aim is to talk freely with the population, monitor the aid chain and reassess the situation as it develops. This is necessary for MSF's teams to make independent judgements. Whatever the situation, it is essential to know which policies the organisation is supporting: thus, although France's policies for excluding migrants have real consequences on their health, they are accompanied by a system of healthcare safety nets that the government encourages NGOs to help it manage. But by treating people without challenging the political and social origins of their exclusion, is MSF not confining itself to the role expected of it by the authorities? In other words, playing into their hands by looking after the people deliberately rejected at the margins of society? This is the question raised in the chapter "Managing the 'Undesirables'", which discusses the way MSF's ambitions have changed regarding its programmes in France.

In extreme situations, MSF's ability to judge is what enables it to keep a distance from "that blurry, but very real, line beyond which assistance for victims imperceptibly turns into support for their tormenters".[8] The organisation's experiences over the years are clear evidence of this, for example, its inability to account for the use of assistance provided to Cambodia in 1980; participation in a lethal policy of forced displacements in Ethiopia in 1985; and the horror of serving as bait and facilitating the work of the executioners in Zaire/ Democratic Republic of Congo in 1996–1997.[9] In such circumstances, the objective for a humanitarian doctor, as Paul Ricoeur reminds us in the book *Médecins tortionnaires, médecins resistants*,[10] is to avoid the "crude [contradiction] between treating a patient and declaring a person sentenced to death to be fit enough to die. [...] It is not through his medical expertise that the doctor will find a way out, but in his moral and political judgement".

But however painful this dilemma may be, it is never posed in such clear terms at the time. The case study on Sri Lanka, "Amid All-Out War", shows how difficult it is for MSF to be sure of its decisions, or even of its observations: isn't the real purpose of the internment camps of the Tamil population to slowly wipe this population out? How can we be sure that MSF's hospital is receiving the most serious cases? Is its hospital not simply being used as a propaganda smokescreen by a government seeking to give an appearance of normality? Are the patients being selected according to their supposed political affiliation? These were the questions raised by MSF, which had become the regime's de facto public health auxiliary.

Keep Silent?

The case studies reveal that, over the years, MSF has often opted to sacrifice its freedom of speech. The organisation decided to keep a "low profile", for example, on the bombings it witnessed in Yemen and chose to keep quiet about the consequences of the war in Sri Lanka. In Myanmar, it also decided to say nothing about the constraints the regime was imposing on it, described in the chapter "Golfing with the Generals".

Does refusing to speak out about violence against civilians mean MSF has lost faith in the impact of its statements? In the chapter, "Silence Heals...", Fabrice Weissman analyses the complex relationship between MSF and its public positioning—aimed at influencing the course of a conflict or health crisis or preventing the misappropriation of aid—in an international context marked by the Cold War, the collapse of the bi-polar world order and the development of international criminal justice and so-called humanitarian wars.

Know Our Place

For MSF, negotiating with actors with whom it shares interests, however temporarily, means being willing to adjust its own plans and ambitions. Unless one party's interests are subsumed by the others, an agreement means compromise. The value of this compromise cannot be gauged from a quick glance at the nature of the allies (army, government, armed groups, "civil society" organisations, etc.); it requires a careful examination of the motivations underpinning it and of the real effects it has on relief efforts. Thus, since 2007, the Pakistani army has been a major hindrance to MSF's attempts to provide care to the victims of the war against the armed opposition (see "The Other Side of the COIN"). However, in the response to the earthquake in Pakistani Kashmir in 2005, it was not only the main relief provider, but also a constructive partner for MSF, as Rony Brauman explains in the chapter "Do Something!".

While in a compromise, "everyone keeps their place; no-one is stripped of their order of justification",[11] a dishonest compromise is "a vicious mixture of plans and postulates".[12] In other words, when MSF seeks the reasons for its actions in justifications (peace, stability, justice, growth, etc.), other than its own, it runs the risk of turning a fair deal into a dishonest compromise. So, as discussed in the chapter "Public (Health) Relations", can the organisation justify organising a mass meningitis immunisation campaign with a negligible medical impact as a tactic for maintaining good relations with the north Nigerian authorities?

Justifying its Choices

How does MSF justify its choices to itself and to others? In the chapter, "In the Name of Emergency", Marc Le Pape presents "a (partial) mapping of the range of choices and justifications actually adopted over the course of MSF's interventions during the decade 2000 to 2010 [without suggesting] a preferred route" which illustrates how the organisation evokes, successively or simultaneously, both its role as a "specific actor" with unique experience and "reputedly universal principles" in an attempt to gain ground.

It seems to us that MSF can only justify its compromises to itself in an ethics of action founded on a principle of medical effectiveness and a refusal to be party to policies of domination.

If, by its actions in a given context, MSF cannot hope "to reduce the number of deaths, the suffering and the frequency of incapacitating handicaps within groups of people who are usually poorly served by public health systems",[13] then the compromises it agrees to are neither justifiable nor acceptable. In this respect, however critical one may be of MSF's intervention in Myanmar, we have to admit that the concessions it accepted—limited intervention zones, restrictions on international staff's access to the population and silence about the regime's oppressive policies—produced results. These can be seen in the number of lives saved by a programme for the large-scale treatment of patients with HIV. On the other hand, MSF interventions in natural disasters show that the "imperative for action", whose premises are challenged by Rony Brauman, has long been at odds with the need to do something medically useful. It was only in 2005 in Pakistani Kashmir, and then in Haiti in 2010, that MSF was finally able to show its practical usefulness, and notably its surgical capacity, in the response to earthquakes affecting zones with a dense urban population and unsound housing, which generated large numbers of casualties.

Refusing to be party to policies of domination is an essential ambition for any humanitarian organisation committed to providing impartial and effective aid. All societies inevitably generate their quota of victims—their excluded populations—groups with no share in society, who are doomed to a violent death or to be deprived of things that are essential to their survival (water, food, shelter and medical care). The civilian populations massacred in Sri Lanka during an all-out war fought in the name of the emancipation of the Tamil people for some and the promise of lasting peace for others, and the populations cut off from assistance or the victims of the bombings in the "war on terror" in Afghanistan and Pakistan, are a reminder that imposing peace, democracy and development always costs lives. In conditions such as these, "humanitarian action is necessarily subversive, since partisans of the established order rarely empathise with those whose elimination they tolerate or decree. In other words, the first condition for the success of humanitarian action is refusal to collaborate in this fatal selection process".[14]

The subversive dimension of humanitarian action, as perceived by MSF, also includes the ability to challenge the norms, priorities and distribution of resources decided by the most influential stakeholders in global health, whose major campaigns and initiatives influence public health policies to suit whatever ideologies are in place at the time. In the chapter "Caring for Health", Jean-Hervé Bradol looks back over forty years of tensions and relations between an organisation of doctors and transnational health policies. He recounts the times when MSF broke away from these policies because of their negative effects on the populations it was working with. It was for this reason that the organisation contested the pauperisation of healthcare for refugees in the 1980s, provided treatment to patients with infectious diseases at a time when public health priorities were focused essentially on prevention and control, and helped develop treatment protocols for people with HIV when governments and the pharmaceutical industry were still recommending leaving them to die.

Through this journey, the conditions of MSF's political autonomy have emerged: an undertaking on the part of practitioners to provide the most effective medical assistance possible to populations who have been excluded due to *raison d'Etat* or market interests. It is to satisfy this undertaking that MSF must justify its alliances, question them, flush out any conflicts of interest and maintain a political watch in order to "recognise, and sometimes anticipate the appearance of [...] favourable circumstances, as this is when the most rapid and profound changes to public health policies can be achieved. Such circumstances can be neither permanent nor artificially induced through advocacy".[15]

Antagonisms

Attempting to bring about changes in public health policy, seeking to take charge of the management of an epidemic, formulating new rights for an excluded population, and denouncing the violence of war in the hope of influencing the way a conflict is conducted are all actions revealing an ambition to manage a population in addition, competition, or parallel with the authorities. What makes it possible to imagine an agreement between MSF and these authorities is their shared interest in the way a population is governed. Thus, "non-governmental policy [does not contest] the legitimacy claimed by those in government [...], nor the interests they serve, but the modalities and effects of their management".[16]

What happens when this shared interest disappears? When the Taliban, routed by the international forces in 2001, or the Afghan warlords, marginalised in a state reconstruction process, no longer seek to govern a population or a territory, but rather to wreak terror and havoc? When, in this new strategy, are humanitarians more useful to them dead than alive? When the Ethiopian government confines MSF to the edges of a war that it is waging against the Ogaden National Liberation Front so that it can conduct its reprisals against the population behind closed doors? When the Sri Lankan government turns a deaf ear to dialogue because it has decided on a military solution for ridding itself of the Liberation Tigers of Tamil Eelam, mercilessly crushing the fighters and sacrificing the 30,000 or so people being used as human shields by the rebellion against the army's offensive? In the kind of extreme situation seen in Sri Lanka, should we replace direct action with a "strategy of roundly criticizing institutions"[17] or abdicate and wait for the order of all-out war to be replaced by one in which humanitarian aid can play its part?

As this book goes to press, MSF is preparing to celebrate "forty years of independence". This slogan may seem misleading as, apart from exceptional and temporary circumstances, in moments of severe disruption, MSF is never given total freedom by authorities who totally abdicate their responsibilities. In fact, not only does it need others to authorise its action, but also to take it over, amplify it, prolong it and help implement it. MSF is permeable to outside influences and ideologies.

Therefore, the issue for MSF is not so much achieving total freedom of action, but being able to choose its alliances according to its own objectives, with no allegiances and no concerns about loyalty. In this respect, it is an unreliable and unfaithful partner. It justifies this liability by the need to identify auspicious openings in the political space and seize opportunities, as is highlighted in the chapter "Afghanistan: Regaining Leverage", which tells the tale of MSF's return to this country in 2008. In other words, if we consider that humanitarian aid is not an exact science but an art, then the essence of this art is to create and maintain the conditions of its existence—to generate interest, make itself useful, identify conjunctures that could be propitious for change—and to be capable at all times of modifying the balance of power, creating a hiatus, permanently maintaining the right conditions for pacific conflict with forms of power that may sometimes be partners, and sometimes adversaries, to our action. At a time when humanitarian actors are questioning their ability to overcome the obstacles they are encountering, we hope that this book will help fuel the debate on their ambitions and the best ways of fulfilling them.

PART ONE

Stories

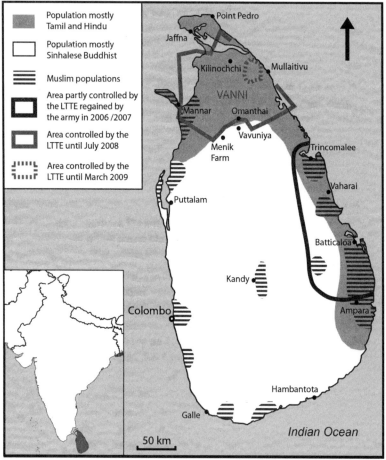

▨	Population mostly Tamil and Hindu
☐	Population mostly Sinhalese Buddhist
☰	Muslim populations
▢	Area partly controlled by the LTTE regained by the army in 2006 /2007
▢	Area controlled by the LTTE until July 2008
⌐⌐⌐	Area controlled by the LTTE until March 2009

Point Pedro
Jaffna
Kilinochchi
Mullaitivu
VANNI
Mannar
Omanthai
Vavuniya
Menik Farm
Trincomalee
Puttalam
Vaharai
Batticaloa
Kandy
Colombo
Ampara
Hambantota
Galle
Indian Ocean

50 km

Sri Lanka

Source: from Le Monde Diplomatique March 2009

SRI LANKA

AMID ALL-OUT WAR

Fabrice Weissman

On 18 May 2009, the Sri Lankan government's crushing victory over the Liberation Tigers of Tamil Eelam (LTTE) put an end to twenty-six years of civil war. Described by the government as the world's largest humanitarian operation, the victorious Colombo offensive was praised as a model by many foreign military commentators[1] keen to demonstrate that a determined democratic army could vanquish a "terrorist" movement. In reality, victory came at the price of thousands of civilian deaths, and the enlisting of humanitarian organisations into a counter-insurgency strategy based on forced displacements and internment. MSF's experience reveals the hard choices that all-out war imposes on aid organisations.

MSF withdrew from Sri Lanka in 2003, after working for seventeen years against a background of civil war between the government and the LTTE that began in the mid-1980s. A ceasefire agreement (CFA) was signed a year before MSF's departure, leading to a return to relative normality and the hope of peace. Negotiations began under the co-presidency of the European Union, the USA and other western coun-

15

tries, including Norway, which also headed a ceasefire observation mission, the Sri Lanka Monitoring Mission (SLMM).

As early as 2003, the discussions stalled on the key question raised by the conflict: how to ensure peaceful coexistence between the Sinhalese, Tamil and Muslim communities, representing 75%, 17% and 8% respectively of the island's population. Although the parties did undertake to explore a federal solution to the conflict, talks became acrimonious once they got down to specifics or tried to agree on a transitional administration for the rebel areas (a third of Sri Lankan territory).[2] A return to warfare seemed imminent when the Sri Lankan coasts were hit by the tsunami on 26 December 2004. Once the emergency response phase ended, management of reconstruction aid rekindled the conflicts over sovereignty between central government and the separatists. In late 2005, attacks, assassinations and abductions escalated in the north east of the country, fuelling a climate of terror. As ceasefire violations increased the eastern provinces slipped into open warfare during April 2006.

From 2006 to 2007, the army regained control of Batticaloa and Trincomalee in the east, driving the LTTE northwards back towards its sanctuary in the Vanni. The following year, the government officially renounced the ceasefire agreement and tightened its grip around the Vanni, taking control of Mannar district in April 2008 before entering Kilinochchi district in July. In January 2009, the army launched its final offensive. The Tigers were boxed into an area of land along the coast that shrank from 300 km² in January to 26 km² in March, 12 km² on 23 April then to 4 km² on 8 May. They were wiped out ten days later and their leader was killed along with most of the political and military commanders.

The LTTE cause most of the ceasefire violations in 2005 to 2006, and was largely responsible for triggering the resumption of hostilities. During the presidential elections in November 2005, it urged the Tamil population to abstain, thus contributing to the victory of Mahinda Rajapaksa, a candidate hostile to the peace process and who narrowly defeated CFA negotiator and former prime minister, Ranil Wickremesinghe. According to Sri Lankan political pundit Jayadeva Uyangoda,[3] the LTTE was then counting on a new confrontation to boost its leverage in future negotiations: a war of attrition would weaken the economy, divide the regime's support base and isolate it internationally due to the war crimes and human rights violations it would certainly commit. Media coverage of the army's violence was in fact the LTTE's main political asset on the international scene.

Even before its official withdrawal from the CFA in January 2008, the Rajapaksa administration made it clear that it was not prepared to negotiate any longer. It used the rhetoric of the global "war on terror" following the events of September 11 2001 to put a security and anti-terrorist spin on the conflict. Denying the existence of the "ethnic problem" at the heart of negotiations and political debate since 1987, the Rajapaksa administration declared the LTTE as the only obstacle to peace, and sought its military and political destruction.

In the face of rapidly advancing government troops, the LTTE dragged tens of thousands of civilians down with them. As the rebel territory shrank, the Tigers used increasingly violent means to dissuade civilians from fleeing to government-controlled areas, executing those that tried to flee and/or making reprisals against their families, and then, in January 2009, strafing, bombarding and launching suicide attacks on columns of civilians trying to reach government lines.[4] Controlling the population was strategically essential to the LTTE for at least two reasons. First, it needed to enlist increasingly younger children to make up for its heavy losses, and second, by mixing fighters with civilians, it forced the government army to choose between two ills: slow down or even halt the offensive, or commit war crimes.

Denouncing the use of the population as a "human shield", in November 2006 the government asked the ICRC and the SLMM to mediate so it could evacuate civilians living in combat zones to camps behind its lines. The Tigers opposed the operation. Colombo then described its offensive as a "humanitarian mission" seeking to "free innocent civilians held hostage by the LTTE".[5]

In reality, although the army claimed to "adhere to the zero civilian casualty (ZCC) policy",[6] it did not let itself be troubled by the presence of aid workers and civilians during its push forwards. Camps for internally displaced persons (IDPs), hospitals, humanitarian convoys and food distribution sites were hit by government artillery and air strikes on several occasions.[7] Several hundred civilians fell victim to shells and bullets between 2006 and 2008, several thousand between January and March 2009, and tens of thousands between April and May 2009. According to unofficial UN figures, 7,000 civilians were killed between January and early May 2009, and 13,000 more in the last two weeks of the confrontation. International Crisis Group (ICG) put the figure for civilian deaths at not less than 30,000 during the northern campaign. The government only acknowledged 5,000 civilian deaths and blamed them on the LTTE.[8]

Throughout the conflict, the government carried out an intensive propaganda war designed to mask the terrible human cost of its offensive. It stated that it was leading a "humanitarian war", thereby justifying its co-opting of NGOs and UN agencies into its pacification policies. From 2006 to 2008, MSF tried in vain to resist. Then, in 2009, it attempted to become a major cog in the military-humanitarian machine in the hope of lessening its brutality.

2006 to 2008: The Government Makes the Rules

From 2006 to 2007, the recapture of the east left at least 250 civilians dead and several hundred wounded, according to local human rights organisations.[9] The fighting displaced 160,000 people. They received various forms of aid from the government, NGOs and UN agencies invited by Colombo to set up in the army's wake, but this only lasted a few months. In March 2007, by cutting off humanitarian aid and using threats, the government—with the support of the UNHCR—organised the forced return of displaced people to their towns and villages, now destroyed and placed under military rule.

The first government victories went hand-in-hand with escalating political violence (abductions, assassinations and threats) targeting Sri Lankan figures who openly criticised the new administration's militarism and xenophobic nationalism. Foreign journalists and international NGOs were also the targets of intimidation. Exploiting Sri Lankan society's distrust of NGOs since their arrival en masse in December 2004, a phenomenon Sri Lankans described as a "second tsunami", the nationalist media regularly accused humanitarian aid organisations of being "war profiteers" and "stooges of the terrorists".[10]

A grenade attack hit three international NGOs in the eastern provinces in May 2006, wounding three people. On 4 August 2006, seventeen Sri Lankan employees from Action Contre la Faim (ACF) were executed in their office in Muttur on the east coast, a few hours after pro-government forces recaptured the town. The assassination, an unprecedented event in the history of humanitarian action in Sri Lanka and for which the SLMM held the government responsible, was officially condemned by senior western diplomats and the UN. The government responded by creating an investigation commission, whose investigations led nowhere. From 2007 to 2009, more than ten humanitarian workers were assassinated, including several ICRC employees.

MSF's Goals

Anticipating a renewal of hostilities, MSF's French section sent several exploratory missions to Sri Lanka in the first half of 2006, which were soon joined by teams from the Dutch and Spanish sections. In July and August 2006, the three sections proposed opening surgical programmes in three hospitals in the government-controlled zone near the front lines in Point Pedro (northern front), Vavuniya (southern front) and Mannar (western front). Their shared objective was to operate eventually in Tiger-controlled zones, with the French section already proposing to open a mission between Batticaloa and Trincomalee on the eastern front, where the first population displacements had been reported.

However, none of the evaluation teams observed any urgent needs. Sri Lanka had qualified personnel and an effective healthcare system, thanks to the ambitious social policies adopted after independence. Furthermore, wishing to assert its symbolic sovereignty over all the national territory, the government had continued to run public services in rebel areas, paying health workers' salaries and ensuring supplies for medical facilities. In addition, a great many humanitarian aid organisations that had arrived in the wake of the tsunami were still in the country in 2006.

In such circumstances, the operations proposed for Point Pedro, Mannar, Vavuniya and in Tiger-controlled territories were primarily about being prepared. MSF sought to expand its healthcare services and emergency response capacity in areas where the organisation expected the conflict to resume with the predictable consequences: a breakdown in medical supply lines, departure of local medical personnel and an influx of wounded and IDPs. MSF's goal, even if not always clearly expressed (except by the Dutch section), was also to ensure an international presence in conflict areas in order to "bear witness to the plight of the population", in the hope of encouraging the belligerents to exercise restraint in the use of violence.[11]

Discord

As the first shells fired by the government's "humanitarian mission" started to rain down on the eastern front in July 2006, the MSF-France teams thought they could obtain the necessary authorisations to launch their activities within a reasonable timescale. They felt that the organisation had acquired legitimacy in Sri Lanka through its presence on both sides of the front line from 1986 to 2003, and its response to the tsunami. By calling a halt to donations three days after the catastrophe, explaining that reconstruction was the responsibility of the state and that most emergency needs were already covered by the authorities and civil society, MSF had flattered national Sri Lankan pride.

The MSF teams soon lost their illusions. Despite support from the local authorities and the Ministry of Health, requests for import licences, visas and authorisations to travel within the country got lost in a bureaucratic maze. As failure followed failure, it became clear that no decision could be taken without the approval of the Ministry of Defence and the president's entourage, whose grip on the state apparatus was tightening.

Starting in July 2006, the Ministry of Defence had indeed restricted access to the rebel zones affected by fighting (designated "uncleared areas") to the ICRC and selected UN agency teams that were only allowed short visits. Other aid organisations had been asked to work in government-controlled zones behind the lines. Failing to negotiate special status, comparable to that enjoyed by the ICRC and UN agencies, the French section decided to exert media and diplomatic pressure. On 9 August 2006, it published a press release denouncing the murder of the ACF workers and the "lack of medical help [for] tens of thousands of people living at the heart of the military offensive". A week later, it organised a series of bilateral meetings with western ambassadors and the peace process co-presidents, feeling that the latter "had the ear of the government". In late August, MSF-France managed to meet with Basil Rajapaksa, special adviser to the president, and Gotabaya Rajapaksa, secretary of defence. Although the president's two brothers assured MSF that it was welcome to work in hospitals designated by the Ministry of Health, they lost their tempers when the head of mission demanded access to rebel zones. MSF was accused of partiality towards the LTTE and of "wanting to tell the government what to do".[12]

MSF found itself in a delicate negotiating position. In August 2006, it had no information indicating that the aid provided by the government, ICRC and UN agencies in the "uncleared areas" was inadequate. MSF estimated that the existing set-up would not be able to cope with the expected influx of wounded and IDPs, an assessment rejected by the government who claimed that the consequences of the conflict would be minimal and handled appropriately by the authorised agencies. In reality, these disagreements masked underlying discord: MSF was keen to use its freedom of speech to denounce the excessive use of force its teams might witness while the government was keen to limit the number of observers likely to reveal the war crimes it was to commit.

Crisis

On 30 September 2006, while head office was encouraging the MSF field teams to stand firm, the French section learned from the national daily press that it was subject to an expulsion order, along with MSF-Spain and five other international NGOs. This was confirmed the same day in a letter from the Department of Immigration ordering MSF teams to leave the country within one week due to "activities […] in contravention of the visa conditions". The press blamed the expulsion on MSF's pro-LTTE commitment: quoting Ministry of Defence sources, it claimed that the organisation had carried out "clandestine activities" for the Tigers under cover of post-tsunami reconstruction aid.[13]

MSF immediately asked for support from the embassies of the expatriates targeted by the expulsion measures. On 5 October 2006, the minister of human rights told MSF that the expulsion order was on hold pending the results of an investigation into its activities. The head of state had just met with the CFA co-presidents and officially declared that he "would continue to facilitate humanitarian access to the conflict-affected areas while keeping in mind security considerations".

Nevertheless, MSF staff still had no work permits and remained publicly accused of pro-LTTE clandestine activities. In mid-October 2006, the heads of mission wondered what they could do to rebuild MSF's reputation when there was little chance of a government retraction. MSF's international president, who had come to support them in the wake of the expulsion, had tried to publish a denial in the local media, calling a press conference in the hope of "clearing MSF's name". Only two (English-language) newspapers reported it.

What safety guarantees should MSF demand from the authorities, the heads of mission asked themselves, when the ICRC had just come under grenade attack a few days after having been accused of pro-LTTE partiality by the press, and the Ministry of Defence had refused to meet with MSF, relegating the crisis to a visa problem that had already been solved. Should they be happy with the suspension of the expulsion order and recent press restraint (MSF-Holland) or demand a public statement of support announcing that proceedings were being dropped and guaranteeing MSF teams' safety (MSF-France) in line with the international president's publicly-expressed position? How long could MSF wait for work permits?

Although all the sections were wondering if they should pull out, only MSF-France seemed determined to put words into action; on 13 October 2006, the head of operations warned: "If we don't see some concrete results soon, we will have to take the decision to leave the country because of the lack of humanitarian space". Not everyone agreed with this option: could they turn their back on the country when all evidence pointed to the conflict being on the brink of escalating? What purpose would be served by one or more sections leaving? Should they simply redeploy their intervention resources to those areas where the organisation was accepted? Or stage a media event to put the government in an awkward diplomatic position and strengthen the negotiating position of the organisations that were staying put?

Compromise

The three sections finally chose to continue to negotiate. They stopped seeking an official denial, the abandonment of the investigation and a public statement of support, and ended up signing a Memorandum of Understanding (MoU) allowing them to launch operations in three hospitals selected by the Ministry of Health. The question of access to "uncleared areas" was not raised. The projects opened in December 2006 and January 2007.

During the two years that followed, the medical-surgical missions in Point Pedro (MSF-France), Mannar (MSF-Spain) and Vavuniya (MSF-Holland) were not over-stretched. In 2007, most of the wounded and people displaced by war were concentrated on the eastern front, while in 2008 the operation to surround the Vanni had not yet caused many civilian casualties. MSF's operations did nonetheless ensure continuity of healthcare (emergencies and surgery) in hospitals with insufficient specialists, dealing with supply breakdowns and the rigours of military occupation. In Vavuniya, MSF-Holland had to suspend surgical activities in March 2008 as the increased Ministry of Health teams made its presence redundant. MSF-Spain decided to close the Mannar programme after the army recaptured the district in late 2008, and left the country the following year.

The French section tried nevertheless to gain access to the eastern provinces where the army was making fast progress. In order to be allowed into the "uncleared areas", it turned to the UN. In late October 2006, the resident UN coordinator endeavoured to negotiate a procedure with the government for designating organisations approved to work in rebel zones and, in November 2006, it obtained authorisation for access from the Ministry of Defence for twenty-one NGOs, one of which was MSF.

Having obtained their passes, the coordination team carried out an evaluation mission in Tiger-controlled areas close to Vaharai in February 2007. However, it did not manage to obtain the necessary authorisations to start up the project before the government forces recaptured the zone a month later, making the planned intervention irrelevant. In April 2007, it proposed providing support to the Batticaloa hospital as the surgical unit was overflowing after the army's recapture of the coastal strip to the south of the town. Once again, Colombo's administrative obstruction and the lack of human resources in Paris delayed the intervention. The surgical teams arrived in August 2007, at a time when the hospital's activities had returned to normal and the eastern provinces were almost entirely pacified.

The French section settled for helping IDPs, providing modest support (mobile clinics, sanitation and distribution of essential goods) to around 30,000 of the 160,000 people caught in the midst of the government's forced displacement/resettlement operation. It closed its programme in January 2008, without ever really looking at the issues raised by its participation in forced population transfers organised with HCR support.

In the end, only the Dutch section managed to set up in Tiger-controlled territories, although it was far from the combat zone. In May 2007, it opened a programme in the LTTE "capital" Kilinochchi which was not yet affected by the fighting. It chose to support the gynaecological, obstetrical and paediatrics units with a view to getting prepared.

But as the front came closer in the summer of 2008, bringing displaced civilians to Kilinochchi, difficult relations with the hospital's medical staff forced MSF to limit its intervention to logistics aid for the waste treatment area and building latrines for the IDPs. On 8 September 2008, the government ordered all the humanitarian aid organisations other than the ICRC and selected UN teams to evacuate the Vanni.

MSF was one of the first organisations to leave the LTTE zones. Its immediate efforts to return encountered a categorical refusal from the secretary of defence, whom they met on 28 November 2008. Asked to pressure the authorities, the Indian and western embassies said they were powerless. Since 2007, Sri Lanka had been drawing closer to China, Pakistan and Iran, with which it had signed a series of economic and military agreements.

After three years of negotiation, as the conflict seemed on the verge of a decisive confrontation that would not spare the civilian populations, MSF had just one surgical programme in Point Pedro, a small-scale project supporting the Vavuniya health district, and very little hope of gaining access to conflict zones. Moreover, MSF was not comfortable with making its voice heard: since the 2006 crisis, it felt that public criticism of the government was likely to lead to expulsion or even physical reprisals against its staff. The MSF teams seemed completely at a loss as to what to do.

2009: All-out War and the Humanitarian Solution to the Tamil Question

Between January and May 2009, the fighting was concentrated on a constantly shrinking and densely populated area and the number of civilian victims increased sharply. In LTTE zones, the wounded had access only to rudimentary care provided by eight Sri Lankan doctors from the Ministry of Health who had refused to abandon their post. The ICRC, which continued to provide them with medical supplies overland then by sea until 9 May 2009, managed to transfer 6,600 wounded and seriously ill people as well as those accompanying them, a total of 13,000 people, to government-controlled areas.

The army evacuated almost 300,000 people from territories gradually recaptured from the Tigers. Soldiers escorted the survivors to transit zones where they were screened: people suspected of belonging to the LTTE were transferred to demobilisation camps, called "rehabilitation centres", and the others to closed internment camps managed by the army and called "welfare centres". Ringed by several rows of barbed wire, the camps were guarded by the army and police.

The largest "welfare centre" was at Menik Farm to the south of Vavuniya, in a marshy and isolated area. Its construction began in September 2008 and was coordinated by the army, which completed the first two zones of the complex. In early February 2009, Colombo asked for help from humanitarian agencies and donor countries in building five additional zones. The medical project included the opening of 1,400 beds in hospitals around the centre and installing five small hospitals and twenty health units within the centres. These "welfare villages" were intended to house 200,000 people for three to five years. Donors were very reluctant to finance construction of permanent internment camps, but ended up agreeing to support the emergency programme for a few months, in exchange for a commitment from the government to resettle 80% of displaced people by the end of 2009.

In February 2009, the announcement of the setting up of Menik Farm stirred up controversy both nationally and internationally, a controversy that grew fiercer in July. Sri Lankan, Indian and British members of parliament compared the "welfare centres" to "concentration camps", reminiscent of those in Nazi Germany.[14] International journalists, who had been banned from going to Menik Farm other than during a handful of guided visits organised by the army, gave wide coverage to alarmist claims about health conditions in the camps. In July, British daily newspaper *The Times* claimed it had been told by senior aid sources that 1,400 people were dying in the camp each week,[15] and added that the death toll lent credence to allegations of "ethnic cleansing" by the government. The press began to question the role of the UN and aid organisations. The UN was accused of "having hidden the scale of the massacres",[16] British aid to war victims was suspected of being used "to fund concentration camps",[17] and the UN and NGOs of being "complicit in a large-scale detention operation".[18]

Waiting in the Wings

Between January and 20 April 2009, MSF watched the crushing of the Vanni from afar. In late January 2009, the first civilians began to arrive in the government-controlled zone, making the Dutch section operational once more. The sick and wounded evacuated from the combat zones began to crowd into Vavuniya's general hospital, where the number of hospitalised patients jumped from 365 to 1,004 between 1 February and 1 April. First one, then another MSF-Holland surgeon came to join the Sri Lankan team. MSF hired nursing auxiliaries to improve post-operative care. But it could do no more: the authorities refused to allow an anaesthetist and two extra expatriate nurses to join the team. They also opposed increasing surgical teams in the other hospitals which were taking in the wounded evacuated by the ICRC.

In Vavuniya district, the dozen internment camps set up in public buildings were soon overwhelmed, leading soldiers to transfer the first interned civilians to zones zero and one at Menik Farm in February. The military and health authorities in Vavuniya asked for support from the UN and NGOs to assist recently evacuated populations. The local authorities were seeking organisations to distribute special food supplements to the under-fives and pregnant and breast-feeding women in the internment centres, and the Dutch section agreed to help. Distribution began in mid-February 2009, despite the lack of any formal agreement from the Ministry of Health in the capital, which had made clear its wish to be the sole provider of medical and nutritional assistance in the camps. "[Local administrators] really want us to bring staff, no matter what they say in Colombo. We also got full access to all camps, and the army general [in charge of supervising the camps] gave us his personal cell number in case anyone objects", reported the MSF-Holland head of mission.

In direct contact with the displaced and wounded coming out of the Vanni, the Dutch section played a part in disclosing the brutality of the regime's counter-insurgency campaign and its internment policies. Between January and March 2009, it issued a press release and posted several updates on MSF websites describing the living conditions of civilians caught up in artillery fire in the Vanni and the lack of freedom for the displaced people interned in Vavuniya. Several MSF representatives talked to the international media about these issues. While the ICRC was claiming that "plain common sense dictate[s] that the civilian population should be urgently evacuated [from combat zones]",[19] MSF "called on all parties to the conflict to allow independent humanitarian agencies to provide medical aid to the wounded in the Vanni".

With activities functioning only in Point Pedro, the French section took a more discreet approach. It limited itself to relaying some of MSF-Holland's information and giving a number of interviews in which it expressed alarm at the bombing of civilian zones and health facilities, a practice already strongly condemned by the ICRC, human rights organisations, the UN and western embassies, which in February demanded a "humanitarian ceasefire" to spare civilian lives.

An Emergency Situation

On 20 April 2009, the army broke through the LTTE's defensive lines and cut its territory in two, triggering the evacuation of over 100,000 civilians in just a few days. The final battle caused an additional 77,000 to be displaced between 14 and 20 May. The evacuated included a great number of wounded. On 21 and 22 April, 400 patients were admitted to Vavuniya hospital, where MSF and Ministry of Health teams operated day and night. In mid-May, the hospital had over 1,900 hospitalised patients, and just 480 beds. As army bulldozers cleared zones 3 to 5, the Menik Farm population rose from under 30,000 inmates to over 220,000 in five weeks. Forty-five thousand people were also interned in small temporary camps in Vavuniya district and 21,000 in camps in Jaffna, Mannar, Batticaloa, Trincomalee and Ampara.

From 20 April the two MSF sections set themselves three priorities: provide emergency care to IDPs in the transit zone, boost operative and post-operative capacity (notably by deploying a field hospital) and develop healthcare provision inside the internment centres. The local authorities, seemingly caught off guard by the scale and speed of the population displacements, proved receptive to most MSF proposals, even asking the Dutch section to open mobile clinics inside the camps "as soon as possible".[20]

In Colombo, the Ministry of Health opposed the proposals. The master plan it had just updated with help from the WHO and UNICEF gave the monopoly in healthcare and public health activities within the camps to the government and carefully selected partners. But Colombo was particularly interested in MSF's proposed interventions outside the internment camps as they fitted in with its plans. On 16 May, the French and Dutch sections each signed a new Memorandum of Understanding with the Ministry of Health authorising them to launch three projects: open a 100-bed surgical field hospital opposite the Menik Farm detention centre (MSF-France), provide additional assistance for treating the wounded at Vavuniya hospital (MSF-Holland), and open a post-operative care unit in Pompaimadhu (MSF-Holland). Faced with an emergency situation, MSF chose to go along with the government's action plans and made two concessions: it renounced, for the time being, negotiating access to transit zones and internment camps, and signed a MoU committing it to "strictly maintain the confidentiality of the information on service provision" and make "no comments [...] without the consent of the Ministry of Health Secretary".

As the programmes approved by Colombo opened in under two weeks, the teams tried to go beyond the authorised activities. When the second wave of IDPs arrived, MSF-Holland succeeded in negotiating at the local level the dispatch of a four-person team to the Omanthai transit zone (where it had tried in vain to intervene in April). From 16 to 20 May, MSF doctors helped with the triage of 77,000 survivors of the final offensive and with boarding them onto army buses heading for the internment camps. The team treated 750 patients, mostly with old wounds that had received little or poor care. All they could do was provide emergency treatment (cleaning wounds, administering antibiotics and pain relief), refer the 200 most serious cases to the hospital at Vavuniya, which they knew was overflowing, and hope that the wounded transferred straight to the camps would receive the care they needed to prevent them from developing crippling and/or fatal infections.

Some of the wounded were transferred to Mannar hospital. The ICRC, which had set up a surgical team in the hospital, reported 800 patients and contacted MSF directly to reinforce its teams. From 23 to 24 May, joint ICRC, MSF and Ministry of Health teams operated on sixty patients with old and infected wounds. But on 25 May as it had not received prior approval from the Ministry of Health, the hospital's management received an order from Colombo to break off cooperation with the ICRC and MSF.

Doubts Arise

Access to camps then became a key issue for MSF. Since the government's "humanitarian mission to rescue civilians held hostage by the LTTE" had turned out to mean carpet-bombing, then would the "welfare villages" turn out to be places where the Tamil population would be left to die?

Access to internment camps was strictly regulated; however, access was possible for national and international staff from MSF, fifty-two

NGOs and UN agencies, except during several forty-eight-hour periods when the security forces carried out screening operations seeking to identify suspected LTTE militants. Even so, MSF was unable to get a precise picture of the health situation. Claiming the monopoly on producing numbers, the government banned any independent epidemiological surveys. The MSF teams had only an approximate idea of health conditions in the camps, based on their visual impressions, brief interviews with internees and longer discussions with hospitalised patients at Vavuniya and Menik Farm. They completed their rough assessment by sharing information with Sri Lankan health workers, national and international employees of other aid agencies, and the security forces, including a number of government officials who openly criticised Colombo's refusal to authorise greater access to the camps for international organisations.

The general impression was that the two huge waves of internees in April and May had created considerable chaos, but that it had gradually been brought under control by the government and aid organisations coordinated by major-general Chandrasiri, the overall head of the internment complexes. The major-general presided over inter-agency coordination meetings and managed aid with an iron fist. In late May, OCHA noted that the camp was short of 15,000 shelters (out of 40,000), that half the latrines had been built and that 75% of water requirements were being met. In private, its representatives acknowledged that the aid services had deployed at an incomparably faster rate than, for example, the slow and chaotic response from the UN and NGOs in Darfur in 2004.

The ministry's master plan seemed to draw straight from public health guidelines drawn up by the WHO and MSF, but the government appeared to have trouble implementing them, despite claiming the enlisting of 300 doctors and 1,000 nurses. The teams learnt from different concurring sources (the police, the morgue and the ICRC in charge of distributing body bags) that the number of deaths at Menik Farm was between ten and fifteen a day in late May. When set against the overall population of the camp, it corresponded to a daily mortality rate of 0.45 per ten thousand and, although this rate was much lower than the emergency thresholds used in Africa, it was three times higher than the national average. The detainees were not dying en masse, but the initial disorganisation of the healthcare system (denounced by some of the Sri Lankan doctors who went on strike in the summer) was in all likelihood the cause of a higher death rate among physiologically weakened inmates, such as the wounded, the elderly, children and those suffering from chronic diseases.

In June, the two MSF sections made several proposals for interventions inside the camps (primary healthcare, nutrition, surgical consultations, mental healthcare, epidemiological monitoring, etc.). They were all turned down, more or less explicitly. This refusal increased the teams' doubts and unease. Why was the government insisting on prohibiting MSF from carrying out any health activities within the camps? Was it trying to mask a serious deterioration in the health situation, or ferocious political repression?

The MSF-France teams working at the Menik Farm hospital were particularly puzzled. No more than 70% of beds were occupied, whereas the other outlying hospitals were still overflowing. With no control over selecting the patients arriving from the camps, MSF wondered what was behind the underuse of its hospital. How could it be sure that the most serious cases were being given priority? Were the patients subject to a politically-skewed selection process? Was the MSF hospital merely a propaganda tool for a government seeking to create the appearance of normality? At the head offices and in the field, many MSF members asked themselves if all the sections should leave the camps and denounce the regime's detention policies, to which aid organisations were public health auxiliaries.

Making a Choice

Following a visit by head office in June 2009, the French section chose to stay put, although they were fully aware of the role the government had assigned them: contribute to maintaining public health order in the internment camps, the main function of which was to monitor and control "dangerous" populations and stifle any fresh surge in Tamil nationalism.[21] Having decreed the abolition of minorities and thereby dispensed with taking their political aspirations into account,[22] the Rajapaksa administration sought to reduce the citizens from the Vanni to beneficiaries of the state's humanitarian benevolence, well-cared for, well-fed, well-housed and, most importantly, well-guarded. The Menik "Farm" symbolised this policy, which extended beyond the barbed wire, as illustrated by the Ministry of Defence's decision to recruit

50,000 extra soldiers after the war was over. This last initiative lent credence to critics of the regime who denounced a pacification of the Vanni in the form of long-term military occupation.

The only concessions that the international actors (states, the UN, NGOs, etc.) could count on concerned the relaxing of the detention policy: transparency of the screening process, release of certain categories of internees and improved detention conditions. Head office felt that MSF should contribute to these improvements. MSF-France therefore sought to become an essential cog in the internment camps' health system: in July, it expanded its hospitalisation capacity, improved its technical services (radiology, ultrasound, laboratories, etc.) and replaced the hospital tents with semi-permanent buildings. It also started to try and get some internees released on medical grounds.

This position was poles apart from the stance taken by other humanitarian aid organisations and donors, particularly the USA and the EU. Funding the camps to the tune of 700,000 dollars a day, in June 2009 the UN and its donors opposed the major improvements in aid standards demanded by the government (construction of permanent shelters and latrines with septic tanks, extension of healthcare infrastructures and the running water network, etc.) so as to underline the temporary nature of the internment camps. During the same period, most NGOs refused to distribute cement to consolidate the floors of the tent and plastic shelters. Yet the housing conditions were precarious. The tents and tarpaulins used throughout the zones (apart from zones 0 and 1 which had permanent structures built by the army) deteriorated rapidly while the latrines overflowed and a foul-smelling tide of mud flooded the groundsheets. In a strange reversal of roles, the government accused aid organisations of causing a "humanitarian crisis" and holding the IDPs hostage to make the authorities give in to their demands. The accusations grew fiercer in August 2009 when the first monsoon rains transformed the camps into open sewers. But images of flooded camps also served as a tool for mobilising opinion and were seized upon by human rights organisations and some Sri Lankan politicians who demanded "a prompt and rapid resettlement of displaced persons to their places of origin".

The decision by General Sarath Fonseka, commander-in-chief of the Sri Lankan army and leader of the victorious offensive, to join the opposition and run against the outgoing head of state in the presidential elections planned for January 2010, had indeed placed the issue of

IDP internment centre stage. Rajapaksa and Fonseka shared the same support base and were trying to attract the minority vote. In August 2009, the former commander-in-chief denounced the fate meted out to internees by the Rajapaksa administration. Combined with international pressure, these electoral concerns persuaded the regime to open the camps and initiate a fast-paced resettlement policy starting in September 2009. By 31 December over half the IDPs had already been sent back to their towns and villages, destroyed, mined and tightly controlled by the army and plainclothes security forces. The French and Dutch sections closed down their emergency programmes. The Menik Farm hospital never became the main hospital for the internment camps. Four thousand admissions were recorded between 22 May and 6 December including 585 suffering from war wounds. According to the information gathered from local health authorities, this 4,000 represented 5% to 10% of all hospitalisations from the camps.

Having returned to Sri Lanka believing that it benefited from a special status in the aid world, MSF found itself in an extremely delicate negotiating position, on a par with the other NGOs. Its weak position sprang primarily from the Tigers' "human shield" strategy of victimisation, which subverted the humanitarian narrative into a propaganda tool to sustain a movement using totalitarian practices. Using the LTTE's treachery as justification, the government showed a remarkable capacity for organising and justifying the subjugation of humanitarian aid organisations to its political and military interests. MSF found itself assigned the role of assisting in a pacification policy that had settled the ethnic question in Sri Lanka by bombings and military surveillance, providing humanitarian aid to populations decreed to be dangerous.

Under permanent threat of administrative obstruction and violent reprisals, MSF did not know how to get the political support it needed to resist. Lacking allies in Sri Lankan society, it looked to western states and the UN, whose influence was waning. MSF ended up accepting the government's diktats, imposing the places, targets and mechanisms for intervention, while counting on bureaucratic flaws in the system and its internal pockets of protest to retain some degree of autonomy. MSF decided not to make use of its freedom of speech to attack a regime that was eager to appear to the world and its own society as the guarantor of a rule of law and democratic values. At the end of the day, MSF adopted a policy of opting for the lesser evil, aimed at improving the condition of survivors of an all-out war that no political power seemed capable of checking.

Translated from French by Nina Friedman

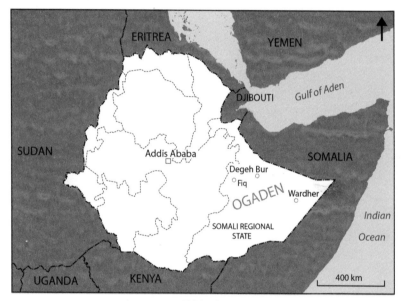

Ethiopia

ETHIOPIA

A FOOL'S GAME IN OGADEN

Laurence Binet

The Ogaden region in the Somali regional state of Ethiopia has been the scene of conflict between the Ethiopian federal government and the Ogaden National Liberation Front (ONLF) separatist movement since 1994. In April 2007, the fighting intensified. After a series of rebel offensives, a wave of repression hit the region, which saw villages attacked and burned, violence and forced displacements, denial of access to wells and a blockade on all commercial traffic, vital to the nomads who inhabit the area.[1]

In 2007, MSF's objective was to provide care for the victims of the conflict. In a region with very few medical facilities and a dispersed population, this meant supporting health centres and organising mobile clinics to go where patients were in need of treatment.

Since the beginning of 2007, the Dutch section's team had been trying to set up a programme in the Wardher hospital on the outskirts of the conflict, but the army regularly denied MSF access to the population living in the area. After a rebel attack near its base in July, MSF decided on a temporary evacuation that was followed by the authorities banning the organisation from returning. Before pulling out, during the few rounds of medical consultations it had managed to hold, MSF had been able to collect witness reports on the acts of violence committed by the warring factions.

During the same period, the Belgian section was prohibited from completing an exploratory assessment at the centre of the conflict zone in the area around Fiq where it was preparing to start up a programme and the ICRC, accused by the Ethiopian authorities of supporting the ONLF, was expelled from the Somali region.

No other humanitarian organisations were active in the conflict-ridden areas of Ogaden. The army's distribution of WFP aid raised questions of impartiality as it was suspected of using the aid to reward people for keeping their distance from the ONLF.

In early September, after a series of diplomatic meetings with Ethiopia's main donors and other stakeholders that brought few results, MSF held a press conference to condemn the government's refusal to allow humanitarian organisations into the Ogaden region.[2] Accounts of human rights violations, documented by the Dutch section, were also cited at the press conference and reported by the international media.[3]

The government then accused MSF of violating its sovereignty and supporting the ONLF.[4] The Belgian section was ordered to close down its long-standing programme for tuberculosis patients outside the conflict zone and the ban on the Dutch team returning to Wardher was maintained.

In the meantime, OCHA, responding to the alerts on the situation in Ogaden, issued in particular by MSF, sent a fact-finding mission which reported a worsening of the health and economic situation in certain areas:[5] difficult access to water and food, shortage of drugs and therapeutic foods, and many cases of acute diarrhoea and measles. In November, OCHA obtained permission from the Ethiopian authorities for several international organisations to work in Ogaden. As the authorities were continuing to block the return of the Belgian and Dutch sections, the MSF movement encouraged applications from the Swiss and Spanish sections that went on to become some of the chosen few. OCHA also obtained the promise that WFP officials could be present when the army distributed food aid, a promise that was not to be kept.

In January 2008, the Swiss and Spanish sections started up medical and nutritional programmes in the areas of Fiq and Degeh Bur that were directly affected by the conflict and the Dutch section returned to Wardher, without authorisation but not officially banned either. But, in reality, by mid-January the operations of two sections were at a standstill. The team of the Dutch section was put under house arrest in Wardher after one of its lorries refused to stop at an army roadblock, and several national staff members were accused of spying for the ONLF. With no explanation, an MSF-Switzerland field team was also ordered to shut down its exploratory mission and forbidden to leave the hotel. Before the mission was suspended, the team had observed that the people it had encountered were victims of violence and suffering from shortages of water, food and medical care due to the restrictions on movement caused by the conflict. However, MSF headquarters was reluctant to draw overall conclusions from these events with regard to the situation in the region as a whole.

In March, the house arrest orders had only just been lifted when all the MSF teams were hindered, on the pretext that most of the expatriate staff members didn't have work permits.[6] In May, a severe nutritional crisis necessitated the assistance of international organisations to conduct emergency relief operations in several Ethiopian states and the authorities took a more relaxed attitude to the question of work permits.

In the Fiq area, however, the MSF-Switzerland field teams were still paralysed and, in June, several national staff members were accused of spying and imprisoned. A month later, the Swiss section shut down its programme and issued a public condemnation of the administrative obstruction that was preventing it from providing relief to the population.[7] It also circulated a document to donors, international institutions and embassies denouncing the Ethiopian authorities' exploitation of emergency food aid for political ends and the absence of a response from the United Nations.[8] The other sections, hoping to be able to work within the limits allowed them and judging that they lacked solid evidence of the misappropriation of aid, did not join MSF-Switzerland in the condemnation.

In the following years, managing as best they could with the endless administrative hurdles, they instigated programmes to support health facilities in areas of ongoing, low-intensity conflict. They provided medical and nutritional aid to the inhabitants—who lacked such care even in times of peace—and medical care to Somali refugees in the transit camps on the border.

Conflicting Objectives

The issue of access to Ogaden in 2007 to 2008 was marked from the outset by a conflict between MSF's goals and those of the Ethiopian government. The latter regarded international humanitarian organisations' aid to the inhabitants of ONLF-controlled areas as potential support for the rebellion. Any contact with the insurgents—even though such contact was crucial to impartial distribution of aid and the safety of the humanitarian teams—was condemned as a sign of political partiality. This position was clearly expressed and defended during meetings with MSF representatives and in the official correspondence sent to them.[9] In 2009, the president of the Somali regional state even confided to a journalist that he believed "that MSF has a hidden agenda. MSF is consulting the 'elders' [clan chiefs] who have close relations with the ONLF, and hiring personnel who support the ONLF".[10]

MSF, convinced of the legitimacy of its cause of providing assistance to the Ogaden people, took a while to realise just how intransigent the government was. It tried to resist the pressure by playing on the fact that there were several MSF sections present and using the levers of diplomatic negotiation and public statement. But those public statements worked to its detriment. The September 2007 press conference referred to the accounts of violence logged by the Dutch section's team, even though they had been regarded initially as insufficiently documented. This increased the Ethiopian authorities' mistrust of MSF, who they accused of spreading propaganda on behalf of the ONLF under cover of providing humanitarian aid. A few weeks later, representatives of MSF were able to experience the government's intolerance of criticism first-hand. During a meeting with the foreign affairs minister, they were shown a file of press cuttings containing all of MSF's public criticisms of the government dating back to its denunciation of forced displacements during the famine of 1985.

In July 2008, the Swiss section's public criticism of the government's refusal to allow access to the area was weakened as the two other MSF sections were still in Ogaden and did not join in the accusation. A paradox that did not escape the notice of the authorities, who publicly accused MSF of "disseminating rumours whose content is clearly at odds with the reality on the ground".[11]

When it came to negotiating with the authorities, even the heads of mission acknowledged that MSF's network of official contacts in Ethiopia was insufficient and poorly organised. The operational teams, often with little experience in the country, struggled to identify the right contacts within a complex governmental system with blurred levels of responsibility; decisions on authorisations and restrictions were taken sometimes at regional level and sometimes at federal level, sometimes by the health authorities and sometimes by the army, without any clearly defined rules.

On the diplomatic front, the team responsible for coordinating the different MSF sections' relations with countries, civil society and international institutions saw that appealing to the African Union would be futile, given Ethiopia's prominent role in the organisation. The team therefore concentrated its efforts on United Nations agencies and western donors who, as providers of aid to Ethiopia, were liable to take seriously the difficulties experienced by the people of Ogaden in gaining access to their aid. But Ethiopia is the United States' main African ally and its partner in the "war on terror", particularly in Somalia where the Ethiopian government plays a leading role in the combat against Islamist insurgents.[12] Most of the diplomats and representatives of those UN agencies present in Ethiopia privately expressed their alarm at the government's refusal to allow access to the area and its misappropriation of aid. While many of them encouraged MSF to voice what they were thinking, none of them seemed to have either the means or the ambition to change the balance of power with the Ethiopian government, a past master in the art of controlling aid.

Over the course of these events, the Ethiopian authorities manoeuvred MSF into waltzing twice round the floor. The first time of the first round began when the Ethiopian government launched a crackdown and denied access to the area from April to November 2007. The second was marked by MSF's diplomatic and public protests, and the third by a spurious opening-up in November, briefly imposed on the Ethiopian government after pressure from the United Nations.

In 2008, events speeded up in the second round. Access was refused for longer, the period of opening-up was no more than brief. The authorities engaged in virtually uninterrupted harassment, paralysing all action by the MSF teams.

If MSF resisted the first waltz, it subsequently bent to the tempo that permitted it to stay at the dance. Since what was to be to date its last public statement on the situation in Ogaden, the organisation has kept a low profile, hoping to improve its relations with the authorities and thereby gain wider access to the region. This strategy is designed to enable MSF to assist the inhabitants should the conflict intensify, but there is no reason to believe that the Ethiopian government will be any more willing to open up the area than it was in 2007 and 2008.

Translated from French by Neil Beschers

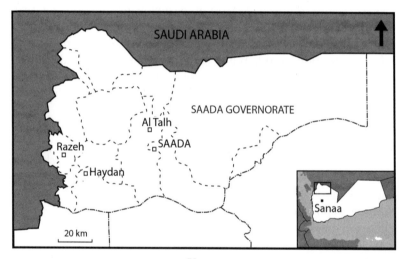

Yemen

YEMEN

A LOW PROFILE

Michel-Olivier Lacharité

In 2004, an insurrection led by former member of parliament Hussein Al Houthi broke out in the northern Yemeni governorate of Saada. His supporters objected to the Yemeni government's political rapprochement with the United States, and demanded the return of Zaydism—the school of Shi'a Islam whose imams ruled Yemen until 1962. Lasting from June 2004 to February 2010, the Saada War was characterised by periods of intense conflict interspersed with relative calm.

The French section of Médecins Sans Frontières conducted an initial exploratory mission in northern Yemen in July 2007, after the signing of a ceasefire a month earlier under the auspices of the government of Qatar. After four episodes of fighting, the government had failed to suppress the Houthist movement, which had failed to gain control of any territory. MSF's objective was to improve access to secondary healthcare in the Saada region, which had few hospitals and was at risk of renewed hostilities with the predictable consequences (war wounded, population displacements, etc.). The organisation started working in Haydan hospital in September 2007, in Razeh hospital in December 2007, and in Al Talh hospital in April 2008. While all three hospitals were in government-held areas when MSF first arrived, they progressively came under Houthi control during the course of the war—Haydan in 2008, and Razeh and Al Talh in 2009.

There was very little media coverage of the Yemen conflict between 2004 and 2007. The lack of war images and reports was due to the Yemeni government's extremely tight control over information, exercised through physical persecution of journalists and legal prosecution of the regime's opponents.[1] These prosecutions stepped up in 2001, helped by Yemeni involvement in the "global war on terror", which signified its alignment with the United States.[2] The government also controlled the communications of the supporters of Al Houthi's movement. Journalists close to the government created a think tank and a website,[3] the analyses of which were aimed at limiting the rebels' capacity for political mobilisation, leaving them with almost no way to get attention, aside from pamphlets distributed to the population and rare contacts with the few journalists who dared cover the conflict.

However, by the time MSF launched its project in September 2007, the situation had evolved over the previous months. Qatar's diplomatic intervention had brought media attention to the conflict—notably by Qatari satellite channel Al Jazeera. The insurgents began distributing DVDs with footage of the war, their military victories and speeches by their leaders, and posted information via electronic mailing lists, allowing them to circumvent the pro-Houthi websites that had been taken down.

MSF was the only international aid organisation to reach the combat zones, aside from the ICRC, which was acting through the Yemeni Red Crescent. One of the few foreign witnesses to the conflict and its disastrous consequences for the population, the organisation faced a dilemma; should it help expose the violence of this little-known war, at the risk of jeopardising its work? Between 2007 and 2009, the shifting context of intervention prompted MSF to choose caution. Its room for manoeuvre depended largely on the goodwill of the government, which required that travel by international staff, drugs and MSF supplies all be approved on a case-by-case basis by the Ministry of Planning, the police, and the governor of Saada. In 2009, MSF deliberately limited its communications to only making its activities in Yemen known locally—in other words, to gaining acceptance from the parties to the conflict.

A Convenient Silence?

Between August 2009 and February 2010, the town of Al Talh came under Houthist control and the hospital where MSF was working found itself on a frontline that advanced and retreated between Al Talh and Saada city. It was hit by bullets and shell fragments on several occasions in August and September.

On 8 September 2009, the MSF hospital teams treated seven children and one woman wounded by the air strikes that hit the centre of the town. Only two of them survived their injuries. On 14 September government planes bombed Al Talh market: thirty-one wounded and nine dead were brought to the hospital. Within moments, Houthist supporters burst in, en masse, to take pictures of the wounded, until MSF teams convinced them to leave by pointing out that the presence of insurgents made the hospital a potential military target. The governmental authority in the region contacted the project coordinator several times that day, assuring her that it had not given the order to bomb, and anxious to know whether MSF was going to say anything publicly about the event. The next day, the central authorities issued a press release in which they denied any responsibility[4] for the air strikes. Two days later, a government plane dropped pamphlets giving the population two options: fight the rebels or leave town.

In the days that followed, the fighting around Saada intensified. MSF teams worried about the impact of the growing insecurity on their ability to continue their work at the hospital. The evacuation routes toward the capital and Saudi Arabia were becoming increasingly dangerous, and the possibility of evacuating the international staff seemed less likely with each passing day. Members of the national staff, who travelled the road between Saada and Al Talh several times a week, were being stopped and harassed by the army, and prevented from moving around. Contacted by MSF in the hopes of obtaining assurances of safety, a high-ranking Yemeni military official advised the organisation to leave. On 22 September, MSF suspended its surgical programmes and arranged to transfer patients to the Saada hospital, about fifteen kilometres away. A few days later the expatriate staff were evacuated from Al Talh, and the national staff left the hospital.

The organisation said nothing publicly about the air strikes it had witnessed, thus failing to honour the commitment that had been made by the MSF movement as a whole in 2006: "We have learned to be cautious in our actions [...] without precluding MSF from denouncing grave and ignored crimes such as the bombing of civilians, attacks on hospitals and diversion of humanitarian aid. Taking a stand in reaction to such situations and confronting others with their responsibilities remains an essential role of MSF".[5] How did MSF justify remaining silent about a serious crime that few direct witnesses relayed to the outside world?

Operational managers at MSF felt that condemning the air strikes would amount to placing blame squarely on the government, and would jeopardise MSF activities in Yemen with little clear benefit. Would speaking out about civilian deaths in the fighting prompt the combatants to show restraint in their use of violence?

More generally, in 2009, MSF was expelled from Darfur, its activities in Niger were suspended by the government and, at the time of the air strikes in Al Talh, a public statement by MSF on internment conditions for people displaced by the Sri Lankan conflict had angered the authorities there. The perceived trade-off between speech and action was being hotly debated within MSF, with some managers demanding that the organisation just keep quiet and deliver care. During an Al Jazeera interview several months earlier in the wake of the Darfur expulsion, MSF's operations director had stated: "You have to be able to distinguish between human rights and international justice activists and relief organisations".

MSF had little desire to risk its entire Yemen operation by denouncing a crime that didn't affect it directly; nor did it want to demand publicly that the warring parties spare the hospital and guarantee the safety of its teams and their freedom of movement. As the fighting intensified, the teams decided to move the staff and patients to safety and evacuate the facility, saying nothing, seeing no immediate tangible benefit to speaking out. On 5 October, however, once the few caregivers who had stayed to receive patients after MSF's departure had all left the hospital, MSF issued a statement to the national press agency and several Yemeni newspapers. Hoping to be able to relaunch its activities in Al Talh someday and fearing the hospital would be looted and bombed, it "called for respect for [Saada governorate] healthcare facilities and their purpose"—in this case, for the deserted building itself and the equipment.

Idle Words

Every year MSF compiled and published its "Top Ten Humanitarian Crises", a public relations effort aimed at increasing its visibility in the media. December 2009 was no exception and Yemen was on the list.

In particular, MSF said that, "Violence escalated sharply in August as Yemeni army forces began carrying out air strikes and artillery assaults against Al Houthi rebels", and reported that "tens of thousands [of civilians fled] into neighbouring Hajja, Amran, and Al Jawf governorates, where they had little to no access to healthcare services".

The information was picked up by Al Jazeera and many other Arab media outlets. The Qatari satellite channel even ran a special edition on MSF's statements on Yemen in December 2009, its analysts wondering publicly about the negative impact this speaking out would have on the credibility of President Saleh.

The government's response was instantaneous. Right in the middle of the war, it immediately suspended authorisation for all of the organisation's activities in Yemen—the movement of people and vehicles, imports, new projects, and the renewal of MSF's framework agreement. In a meeting, government representatives laid out their main grievances to the head of mission: MSF had failed to remain neutral in the conflict by only condemning military violence and not that committed by the Houthists, and it had offered an unfounded evaluation of the healthcare services in government areas where it worked little, if at all. One of MSF's government contacts concluded, "It was this kind of purely political report that got you expelled from Darfur".[6]

Yet listing Yemen as one of the Top Ten Humanitarian Crises served no clear political or operational objective—other than "to attract media attention to a neglected crisis".[7] That lack of intention and objective resulted in a vague description of the conflict and its consequences in which the government may have seen a kind of empathy with the insurgents' cause. And the brief account did present the government as the main culprit in escalating hostilities and impeding aid, cracking down on an uprising "claiming social, economic, political, and religious marginalisation".

The authorities were explicit regarding the terms of the negotiation: if MSF agreed to deny that the Yemeni government was creating problems of access and that there was a lack of healthcare services in government zones, and to stress that the media's sole use of the Yemen case out of the Top Ten report reflected that same media's viewpoint only, the government would lift the sanctions. MSF accepted the deal. In December 2009, MSF operational managers sent the Yemeni government a letter acknowledging that the report may have appeared biased, and that the issues with civilian access to healthcare services were not sufficiently documented. The national press agency issued two press releases with headlines that spoke for themselves: "MSF apologizes for 'inaccurate' report on Saada", and "MSF: apology to Yemen for wrong report on the health conditions of IDPs". These were texted to a number of Yemeni mobile phone subscribers and picked up by about twenty national media organisations and a few international news agencies. The government immediately lifted all sanctions against MSF.

When Al Talh was being shelled, MSF saw speaking out publicly as a threat to its operations, rather than as a way to pressure the government to guarantee the safety of civilians and aid teams. It would have been difficult for the government to challenge immediate and first-hand testimony by a medical organisation treating the civilian victims of the air strikes, and itself affected by the lack of safety. But the Top Ten episode—which proved how sensitive the Yemeni government was about its media image during the war—showed how vulnerable MSF can be when it speaks out without a clear political or operational objective. At that point, the association had nothing to bring to the showdown with the national authorities. It had given the government fodder for its propaganda by denying that there were problems with access to care—problems for which both the government and the rebels were to blame.

Translated from French by Nina Friedman

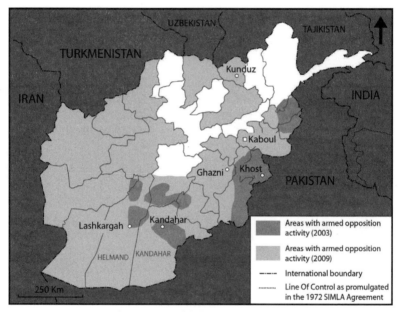

Afghanistan

AFGHANISTAN

REGAINING LEVERAGE

Xavier Crombé (with Michiel Hofman)

On 28 July 2004, two representatives of MSF held a press conference in Kabul to announce the organisation's decision to pull out of Afghanistan. They explained that on 2 June five MSF aid workers had been assassinated in Badghis province and, almost two months on, the Afghan authorities in Kabul had made no attempt to arrest and prosecute the identified suspects. In addition, an alleged Taliban spokesman had claimed responsibility for the killings and justified further attacks by accusing MSF of "spying for the Americans". These facts had led the agency to conclude that "independent humanitarian action, which involves unarmed aid workers going into areas of conflict to provide aid, has become impossible" in Afghanistan.

Although these were the main reasons for the withdrawal, the MSF spokespersons also made clear that the international forces had to share the blame for the deleterious context in which those recent events had taken place. The US-led Coalition's systematic attempts to co-opt humanitarian aid and use it to "win hearts and minds", they claimed, had seriously compromised humanitarian aid workers' image of neutrality and impartiality.[1]

To many of those attending the press conference and who recalled MSF's twenty-four years of presence in Afghanistan—including through some of the worst times the country had known—the decision came as a surprise. "Aren't there ways for you to stay [...] and deal with the security situation?" someone in the audience asked.[2]

In an article published in *The Wall Street Journal* a few weeks later, Cheryl Benard, an American scholar close to the Bush administration, had a ready solution to offer:

It's a different world out there [...] The principle championed by Doctors Without Borders—that civilian professionals providing medical help to the suffering will be granted safe passage—is now part of our nostalgic past [...] An objective assessment of the facts would lead organizations like Doctors Without Borders to demand more military presence, not less; closer cooperation with the military, not a separation of spheres. Alternatively, they will have to withdraw not just from Afghanistan, but also from most of the conflicts of the 21st century.[3]

"In the 'war against terror', all factions want us to choose sides", the president of the International Council of MSF fired back. "Ms. Benard's 'objective assessment' [...] is merely another example of this logic. We refuse to choose sides".[4] The controversy was not new. It had been raging ever since the Bush administration had launched Operation Enduring Freedom (OEF) in Afghanistan in retaliation for the September 11 attacks on American soil and had called on humanitarian NGOs to join in the war effort. Yet, in the months that preceded the killing of its personnel, MSF found itself in an ambivalent position where the western forces and Afghan authorities it wanted to distance itself from were, in effect, its main interlocutors. While opting out of the reconstruction plan designed by an "international community" in open support of the Karzai government, MSF had had no contact with the armed opposition since the fall of the Taliban regime and had considerably reduced its programmes, including in those areas where the insurgency was reportedly gaining ground. The legitimacy that many at MSF felt they deserved, given the organisation's twenty years of history in Afghanistan, was not enough to secure respect for a "humanitarian exception" increasingly at odds with the agenda of the main political, military and aid players on the Afghan scene.

What made it possible then for MSF to return to Afghanistan in 2009 and relaunch programmes, not only in Kabul, but also in Helmand province, one of the areas most contested by western troops, the

Afghan security apparatus and armed opposition groups? The deadliest year for aid workers had been 2008, and 2009 saw civilian and military casualties reach unprecedented levels. In short, there had been no magical re-opening of the "humanitarian space". Yet, the "different world out there" had grown to have implications quite opposite to those asserted by Cheryl Benard only a few years previously. As this chapter argues, the evolution in the dynamics of the conflict and the interests of the various players in Afghanistan have contributed to re-establishing the relevance of MSF's services, granting it renewed leverage to negotiate access to people caught up in war.

Unlike usual representations of humanitarian action—associated with emergency intervention and rapid deployment of resources—the following account shows the ongoing process of reinserting MSF into the Afghan field to be a long and sustained effort to identify and engage negotiating interlocutors on all sides and at all levels along their respective line of command.

"A Different World Out There?"

The most obvious change in the wake of September 11 was that, after years of neglect, Afghanistan was to become the theatre of major and direct intervention by western armed forces. Initially MSF did not have much to say about the US-led OEF, endorsed by the United Nations in the name of legitimate self-defence. As several voices in the international MSF movement stated, the role of a humanitarian agency is not to judge the reasons or objectives of a war, but rather the means used to carry it out. In this respect, the Bush administration's rhetoric of "infinite justice" and "war against terrorism", its reference to NGOs as a "force multiplier" for the US army[5] and its rejection of the applicability of international humanitarian law to "enemy combatants", soon caused concern. In the first phase of the war, however, calls for restraint and respect for the distinction between military and humanitarian responsibilities[6] carried little weight. All the more so as MSF, like most humanitarian agencies, had all but evacuated Afghanistan before the start of the US bombing campaign when the Taliban regime warned it could no longer guarantee the safety of foreign aid workers. Further undermining the relevance of the humanitarian voice at that stage, the expectation of a refugee crisis and of the subsequent emergency needs that had led to massive deployments of aid at the borders of the country proved unfounded.

When, in November 2001, MSF expatriate teams returned to Afghanistan only days after the fall of the Taliban government and the seizure of Kabul by the Northern Alliance, there was no significant emergency situation to address. And, when a few weeks later reports emerged of alleged war crimes by the US army and its Afghan allies—notably the bombing of Taliban prisoners in the prison of Qala-e-Jangi—the MSF movement did not set itself apart from the international community's muted reactions. No consensus could be reached between those who considered a public denunciation of these crimes to be part of the organisation's legitimate role and those who feared it would be seen as overly political, particularly as no humanitarian worker had actually witnessed the events.[7]

Over the following year, the MSF sections that had been present in Afghanistan prior to the Coalition's intervention resumed most of their previous programmes as security conditions allowed. With operations in fifteen provinces by the end of 2002, the MSF movement could again claim to be one of the leading healthcare providers in the country, as it had been for most of the previous decade. However, the implications of such a role were soon to become a problem. With funds now available from a variety of state donors anxious to show their contribution to the American effort, the aid community began to soar. The United Nations agencies were now under the authority of the UN Assistance Mission to Afghanistan (UNAMA) headed by Lakhdar Brahimi. The country was to be the test case for the new integrated approach to UN peace operations that Brahimi himself had played a leading role in designing. Politics and aid were now integrated into the same structure, with politics firmly in the driving seat. This soon translated into an endorsement of the Coalition's military objectives and a requirement that the aid programmes serve the goal of strengthening the legitimacy of the new Afghan government which had emerged from the December 2001 Bonn Agreement.

For the main donors—the United States, the European Commission and the World Bank—health was a prime locus of political legitimacy and a multi-million dollar programme was established in 2003 to allocate the provision of basic healthcare in rural areas of entire provinces to NGOs selected by the Afghan Ministry of Public Health (MOPH) and international donors. The health programme, consistent with the general shift of donor funding towards long-term reconstruction aid, signalled the political will to portray Afghanistan as a "post-conflict" environment. The US army had already delivered this message in November 2002 when it announced the creation of Provincial Reconstruction Teams (PRT), mixed civil-military units "designed to improve security, extend the reach of the Afghan government and facilitate reconstruction in priority provinces".[8] While the aid community, which by mid-2003 amounted to 200 international NGOs and private companies and 800 Afghan organisations, for the main part rejected the PRT's offer to coordinate their actions, most of them readily signed up to the donors' scheme which effectively made them "implementing partners" of the Kabul administration in return for funds.

MSF Leaving Afghanistan: No Compromise Possible

Disbelief was probably the overwhelming feeling of the MSF teams at the time, regarding both the "post-conflict mood" of the international stakeholders and the stated ambitions of development health policies that combined de facto privatisation with bureaucratic control by weak government institutions. Refusing publicly to participate in the reconstruction-funding scheme, they declared instead that the ongoing conflict involving international forces, whether part of the US-led Coalition or the UN-mandated International Security Assistance Force (ISAF), justified the sustained provision of independent and impartial humanitarian assistance.

Although the five MSF sections were united in this position of principle, they were less consistent in translating it into operational terms. By then, most of their programmes were located in relatively stable areas in the centre and north of Afghanistan where they met with the typical uncertainty, associated with "neither war nor peace" situations, as to what distinguished humanitarian medical aid from development-oriented health projects. Throughout 2003 and early 2004, a number of MSF-supported health facilities were handed over to other NGOs or officially to the Afghan Health Ministry. At the same time, MSF attempted to identify what were termed "unaddressed medical needs", such as tuberculosis or malaria, in an effort to retain a useful medical role on the sidelines of the national health policies. Limited in size, such programmes were no doubt of value to their direct beneficiaries, but were of little interest to the Karzai administration and its international backers who were bent on demonstrating quick results on a large scale.

While weakening its position vis-à-vis the Afghan government, MSF's operational choices could hardly appeal to the armed opposition and convince it of the agency's neutrality. Despite maintaining medical programmes in the southern cities of Kandahar and Ghazni, MSF had little visibility or impact on the effects of the relatively silent war building up in the surrounding areas. In fact, it had made no real attempt to restore contact with the Taliban since their fall from power. The murder in Uruzgan province of an ICRC delegate ordered by a Taliban commander in March 2003 made that option even harder to envisage and contributed a few months later to MSF's decision to withdraw its expatriate staff from Ghazni. But the Taliban were not the only threat hanging over humanitarian organisations: they were also easy targets for disgruntled warlords acting as "spoilers" to assert their power and influence and this, in all evidence, accounted for the assassination of the MSF personnel in Badghis province. In spite of all the arguments put forward at the press conference to justify its departure from the country, the killing was felt by many within the MSF movement to be a tragic conclusion to an ongoing process of retreat.

It was, in fact, not the first time the relevance and viability of the organisation's operations had been called into question in Afghanistan. The significance of MSF's cross-border missions in the country in the 1980s was based on a powerful symbol: the "French doctors" were one-sided in their public denunciation of the Soviet occupier's war crimes and the medical aid provided to populations in areas controlled by the mujahedeen displayed solidarity with their cause. Jihad party leaders and local commanders granted the MSF teams protection in return for the assistance they provided to their constituency and for the financial and military support from western states some of them hoped the visible presence of MSF would favour. With the Soviet Union gone and vast US funds having spurred corruption and rivalry among party leaders and the hundreds of aid agencies present in the refugee camps in Pakistan,[9] the pertinence of the small MSF medical teams started to fade. Amid growing disagreements within the organisation over the nature and impartiality of its operations, tensions with mujahedeen escorts[10] and security incidents escalated until the murder of an MSF expatriate in a clinic in Badakhshan province led to the closure of all programmes in Afghanistan in 1990.

When MSF returned after the fall of the communist regime in 1992, it addressed a very different context with very different means. Initiating operations in Kabul, now the scene of an all-out civil war among the different factions, the organisation was able to make use of the logistical capacity developed during the previous decade in other settings—cars, radios and the airlifting of medical supplies. Size of operations mattered more than symbols at the time and it was the presence of three to four MSF sections across the country's multiple frontlines that enabled the organisation to earn its reputation and acceptance. Yet, in early 2001, the relative peace imposed by the Taliban and the destitution in the country, submitted to harsh rule and international sanctions, led to growing unease regarding MSF's continued presence.

An Invitation to Return

Between 2004 and 2008, two significant developments opened the way for some in MSF to reconsider options for a return to Afghanistan. Firstly, it was not long before the "post-conflict" success story started to unravel. Over-confident and anxious to reallocate forces to Iraq, the Bush administration unilaterally decided to reduce US troops in the south and called on its ill-prepared NATO allies to take over. This was the opportunity for the armed opposition based in Pakistan to launch a major offensive in the spring of 2006.[11] In their heartland, the various arms of the Taliban were able to build on the population's growing discontent with the corruption of the government and its local officials, the lack of effective public services in the provinces and resentment against the foreign presence. Their influence gradually extended to other parts of the country, including the north.[12] The international forces' response relied heavily on aerial bombing, resulting in high death tolls among civilians and still further alienation. As revealed in a UNAMA human rights report, civilian casualties caused by armed opposition groups in 2008 only slightly outnumbered those caused by "pro-government forces", two-thirds of which were due to air strikes. That same year, thirty-eight aid workers were killed and 147 kidnapped, leading the UNAMA to conclude that "humanitarian space had shrunk considerably".[13] The report signalled a belated realisation by the UN and aid groups of the price being paid for their years of association with the post-conflict agenda of these same "pro-government forces".

Secondly, and in opposition to the first development, the ICRC had undertaken, during the same period, a unique endeavour to restore dialogue with the armed opposition and to gain recognition of its neutrality. The assassination of its delegate in 2003, followed a few months later by the murderous attack on its delegation in Iraq, had led to much soul-searching within the ICRC. In 2004, while MSF was deciding to withdraw from Afghanistan, the ICRC instead began to make use of the wide range of activities included in its mandate, such as access to detainees, orthopaedic programmes and donations, to demonstrate its operational relevance to the opposition and open up channels of communication with its leadership. The ICRC's approach received its first public recognition in August 2007, when the Taliban granted the organisation a mediation role in the negotiations leading to the release of South Korean hostages.[14]

It was right in the middle of this hostage crisis that an MSF team carried out an assessment in Afghanistan. Its findings conveyed the sense that innovative approaches were needed if MSF was to return to the country. Given the context, the standard practice of having several autonomous sections in the field and programmes run by expatriate staff prone to a high turnover was cause for concern, but much uncertainty remained among MSF sections over what an acceptable alternative could be. With the war now in the open, internal discussion gained momentum in 2008, thanks to a large extent to the ICRC's readiness to share its experience with MSF and facilitate the organisation's return through contacts and advice. The armed opposition appeared to be asking for increased medical assistance for its combatants and the people in the war zones, and the ICRC wished to have other humanitarian actors in the field to help meet the growing needs stemming from the conflict. For MSF to gain credibility with the opposition, ICRC delegates warned, its operations must reach a "critical mass", but having several sections and representations as in the past might jeopardise the ability to develop a reliable network of contacts.

Despite persistent security concerns, these recommendations and offers of support helped to strengthen the case for a return within MSF. There was now a consensus on the necessity for a single representation and, to this end, it was the Belgium section of MSF that was selected to conduct negotiations and assume full operational responsibility in Afghanistan on behalf of the movement for a period of two years. At the same time, preliminary contacts were made with representatives of the armed opposition over the course of 2008, during which the Taliban denied responsibility for the Badghis murders. Although the level of authority and influence of these contacts was still unclear, they seemed to confirm the ICRC's analysis that the armed opposition was now seeing more potential benefits in securing access to medical aid for themselves and their social base than in preventing it. It was now up to the designated operational team to develop a pertinent humanitarian role for MSF in Afghanistan.

Finding Common Ground with the Afghan Government

The broad outline of the operational strategy was set out in February 2009, at the end of a ten-day visit to Kabul led by the newly appointed head of mission. He recommended that the mission be geared toward providing medical care in areas where the health system had been the most disrupted by the conflict. In spite of the lack of reliable data, the war-torn areas in the south and east of the country appeared to be most in need, but accessing them could only be seen as a medium-term objective. Security conditions made travel by road to these areas all but impossible—not only for expatriates but also for Afghans from other parts of the country—let alone conducting health assessments. From the political point of view, these assessments risked being perceived as undermining the Kabul government's authority. According to the official line supported by the international donors and their "implementing partners", the primary healthcare funding programme was now successfully covering 85% of the country's rural districts, a figure based on funds disbursed rather than on effectively running health facilities. It was therefore preferable for MSF to opt for less sensitive operations as a first step to gaining credibility and to develop a reliable local network that would help achieve its longer-term goal. The head of mission recommended focusing on improving secondary healthcare in towns either close to conflict zones or accessible by plane. This would respond to an obvious medical need, since the hospitals in many provincial capitals, and even Kabul, had largely been excluded from donor funding, and it would enable expatriate teams to be sent to the field. The presence of expatriates, albeit limited in number and confined to their accommodation and places of work, was deemed necessary to ensure effective monitoring of the activities but, above all, to conduct direct negotiations with the warring parties, as recommended by the ICRC. "As expectations are high from all sides it will be important to have 'something to show for' reasonably quickly, but also clearly aimed at different parts of the country and different populations", the head of mission noted in his report.[15]

It was thus decided that MSF would support two public hospitals. One was Boost provincial hospital in Lashkar Gah, the capital city of Helmand province, a region where intense fighting had been taking place for several years between the international forces, the Afghan army and the armed opposition; the other was a district hospital in the east suburb of Kabul, an area which was drawing a growing number of migrants and displaced people. By opting for existing public health structures rather than setting up independently-run MSF facilities, the organisation's coordination team hoped to facilitate the negotiation process with the Kabul government on which it depended for visas, work permits and authorisations to import medical equipment, allowing MSF to start operations quickly. As Helmand province was the stronghold of the insurgency and MSF's opposition contacts had expressed an interest in setting up medical programmes in Kabul, it was assumed the two locations could appeal to both sides in the conflict.

As for the Afghan government, political timing played in MSF's favour. Since its departure, the authorities had drawn up new regulations with the tacit support of the UNAMA and international donors to strengthen their control over the NGO community. The NGOs involved in medical activities now had no alternative but to become subcontractors of the Ministry of Public Health (MOPH), through which donor funding was channelled. Yet, with the upcoming presidential election scheduled for the summer and his position at stake, the minister of health saw in MSF's planned operations a way to improve his image. He was therefore willing to exempt the organisation from the subcontracting framework and to press other government departments to legally register MSF in the country. The Memorandums of Understanding (MoUs) for the projects were the subject of little discussion and both were signed on 30 June 2009. The Afghan press agency reported the event in two separate press releases, which left little doubt as to the different positions of the two signatories. In one of them, the minister of health was quoted as saying: "We invited MSF to resume activities in Afghanistan and assured them the government will provide every facility and opportunity to it to implement the [national] strategies".[16] The other one, actively solicited by MSF to counterbalance the MOPH's public relations exercise, cited the head of mission: "MSF will rely solely on private donations, thus safeguarding its independence from political and military powers".[17]

The provisions of the two MoUs gave MSF control over its medical activities and stipulated the application of humanitarian law within the healthcare facilities. While it was agreed that MSF would provide medical assistance "in support of" the MOPH in the two hospitals, drugs and equipment were to stay under MSF supervision right to the patient and all services were to be provided free of charge. Weapons were prohibited within hospital compounds, which from then on would be under the control of MSF-employed guards. Any third-party support for the hospital, notably by international forces, was to be subject to prior agreement. Lastly, in keeping with the Geneva Conventions, patients were not to be harassed or arrested by security forces during treatment and, as long they were not deemed medically fit, to be subjected to interrogation. As for the medical staff, they could not be prosecuted for treating patients, whoever they were.[18]

Disarming International Forces in Health Facilities

Enforcement of these clauses entailed further negotiations, however, especially in the case of Boost hospital in Lashkar Gah. British troops from the ISAF (International Security Assistance Force), private security companies protecting British government development officials, the police, the army and the Afghan secret services—the National Directorate for Security (NDS)—were used to moving around freely and heavily armed inside the hospital premises. While the MoU was effective in getting the Afghan police and army to put a stop to the practice, the others would only comply if ordered to do so by their hierarchy.

Negotiations with the international forces thus started by establishing contact with the British authorities. The coordination team initiated the process in Kabul through meetings with the British ambassador before going to London to meet with the relevant interministerial and military departments. These negotiations enabled MSF to obtain the suspension of the PRT's activities and the definitive withdrawal of soldiers from the hospital. Then, in August 2009, MSF's US-based section set up a series of meetings with US officials from the State Department in Washington and the US military Central Command (CentCom) in Florida. The objectives of the MSF delegation were to inform the US political and military leadership of the medical programmes it planned to develop in Afghanistan and to request that all military forces under US command, including Special Forces, respect the protected status of the MSF medical mission. At the time of the visit, the still-new Obama administration was preparing a second strategic review of the war in Afghanistan. General McChrystal, appointed commander of US and NATO forces in Afghanistan in June, was finalising his assessment of the situation, which was rumoured to be grim. For all that, the US government's public relations policy towards NGOs seemed to have changed little since 2001. In April 2009, Richard Holbrooke, United States special envoy for Afghanistan and Pakistan, had claimed "90% of US knowledge about Afghanistan lies with aid groups"[19] and at the beginning of August, General Petraeus had promoted a new "Civil-Military Fusion Centre"[20] to a panel of UN diplomats and NGOs in Geneva. Nonetheless, State Department and CentCom officials did recognise MSF's need for security guarantees from all the parties to the conflict. In sharp contrast with the usual reactions from the PRT officers in the field, they made no objection to the remark made by the representatives of the organisation that, from a humanitarian perspective, MSF made no difference between its relations with the US military and with the Taliban.

The meetings did not result in any formal commitment, but MSF's objectives appeared to have been met in the field. In the autumn of 2009,[21] ISAF troops raided several health facilities run by international NGOs, but no such incident has taken place in MSF-supported hospitals. The international negotiations may have incidentally led to other benefits. In October, the NDS general in Helmand informed the head of mission that he had received new instructions from Kabul and ordered his staff "to start application of international humanitarian law in Boost Hospital", before adding "the hospital should be a safe place for all patients, whether they are associated with the opposition or not".[22]

Engaging with the Opposition

Full compliance with MSF's "no weapon" policy was to be the starting point for the medical programmes. They were launched officially in Kabul in October, but remained effectively on hold in Lashkar Gah until January 2010. The teams were on the wards, but had to wait for drug supplies to arrive as their transport by truck from Kabul to Helmand depended on obtaining permission from the Islamic Emirates of

Afghanistan (IEA), the most influential armed opposition group, also known as "Quetta Shura". This was in essence a sovereignty issue, as most districts in the southern provinces, and consequently road traffic, were under effective control of this group.

Since MSF's return to Afghanistan, there had been several setbacks in engaging the Taliban leadership. Getting approval for the Kabul project had been relatively straightforward as MSF's initial opposition contacts judged the selected hospital located in a Pashtun area to be easily accessible by their constituency, and planned surgical activities opened up the prospect of treatment for their wounded combatants. But the scant interest and commitment they had shown from the outset regarding MSF's intended projects in the southern provinces, including Helmand, known to be the heartland of the IEA, had cast doubts over the breadth of their connections.

Hence, in the spring of 2009, MSF set about establishing different contacts with the opposition, this time relying on its own network of former Afghan staff and, by the summer, had been able to initiate communication with known IEA members. Right from their first discussions, these new interlocutors made clear to MSF that its earlier contacts were not legitimate representatives of their group. Their connections lay instead with the Haqqani Network, whose influence extended over Kabul and Afghanistan's southeast, as well as the Waziristan region in Pakistan. The IEA was rooted in the south but was also influential in the rising insurgencies in the west and north. The two groups were partner organisations, but they had distinct constituencies and interests. From then on, the two channels should be engaged separately for negotiation, depending on the area at stake.

While MSF had been successful in expanding its network, time had nonetheless been lost in identifying the right contacts to secure guarantees in Helmand. Moreover, soon after a first and promising encounter, the organisation was informed that the IEA council had rejected its two projects, on the grounds that working in MOPH facilities displayed unacceptable support for the Karzai government, derisively referred to as the "Labour Department" of the American forces. This decision effectively prohibited the safe transport of drugs by road from Kabul to Helmand.

It took six more months to resolve the issue. MSF defended its operational choice as a necessary first step to import drugs and insisted that, with its teams already on the ground and drugs waiting in Kabul, it was too late to cut the project short. Assessments for future projects, MSF argued, would consider areas suggested by the IEA. The agency also stressed it had received assurances from foreign and Afghan forces that they would not interfere in the hospitals. On the part of the IEA, security considerations were inseparable from issues of legitimacy and the authorisation for the transport of drugs MSF was asking for was used as a bargaining chip to extract further guarantees and concessions from the organisation. Airing their distrust of the MOPH doctors in Lashkar Gah and of US respect for the Geneva Conventions, the opposition demanded that MSF give a commitment in writing stating that it had control over the hospital staff and provide an official MoU with the US military to prove their compliance with humanitarian law. MSF was careful not to commit itself regarding the behaviour of the international forces, stressing instead its ability to hold them to account through the media.

In January 2010, the IEA eventually gave permission for the drugs to be transported to Helmand. Wishing to be recognised as an able and legitimate government in the regions where they were gradually gaining control, the opposition leadership was seemingly more interested in medical aid as a tool to win "hearts and minds" than as an actual asset for their combatants. When MSF asked if the IEA had suggestions for future projects, one representative answered: "The biggest needs are with civilians, especially maternity care; we can take care of our fighters".

Improving the Quality of Care

The launching of medical activities didn't mean negotiations were over for MSF. At Boost hospital, they were now held on a daily basis between the expatriate team and the local medical staff. Prior to the organisation's arrival, the doctors and nurses had used the provincial hospital as a waiting room for their own private clinics in Lashkar Gah. Even if they hoped to benefit from MSF's support of Boost, many of the provisions they had agreed to during the MoU negotiations in Kabul went against their own business interests, which were potentially threatened by the drugs and treatment now available free of charge at the hospital. The MSF team's effort to organise fixed working hours to ensure continuity of care for patients also created tension as the local doctors resisted being kept away from their highly profitable private practices. These habits and vested interests were hard to change, to the detriment of the quality of care. Negotiations on setting up good management of the hospital were all the more difficult to conduct during the early stages of the project as, in a dangerous environment where MSF was a newcomer, the expatriate team was small and could not take the risk of alienating the local medical team.

By the end of 2010, the mission coordinators considered they had enough guarantees to expand the international medical team in Lashkar Gah. MSF's credibility with the population and the local armed groups required rapid improvement in the services provided by the hospital, all the more so as the issue of quality of care was compounded by that of access. In November 2010, a patient survey concluded that the majority of people in Helmand could neither afford nor risk going to Boost hospital for treatment. Taking a taxi from the districts to the city cost an average of 100 dollars and mines, fighting and intimidation were constant threats that few people would risk, even in cases of dire emergency. The high profile operation carried out by international troops in Helmand province in the spring—part of the "surge" decreed by the Obama administration—had obviously done little to improve the situation. "We're between two forces", one man complained to the survey team, "the Taliban say don't go out at night, the British army patrol checks us during the day". An old man from the Taliban-controlled district of Nawzad was recorded as saying, "They will not stop their fighting for our patients. They are killing each other by the hundreds, why would they stop for just one patient?" Commenting on Boost hospital, he added: "I don't see any weapons here—that means you don't have any problems with the Taliban". Statements such as these came as an endorsement of MSF's approach; they also confirmed the necessity for the team in Lashkar Gah to develop contacts with local opposition leaders in order to gain access to those districts thought to be most affected by the conflict. But as the old man interviewed in the survey concluded: "The Taliban is not under one command. It might be all right for you to be here, but can you come to my district?"[23] Indeed, divisions among opposition commanders in Helmand have up until today prevented MSF from getting the agreements and security guarantees that would allow it to do so.

Scaling Up

A common downside of supporting public structures, the operational difficulties encountered in Boost hospital in Lashkar Gah did not come as a surprise to the mission's coordinators. They had resigned themselves to this option in order to be able to secure the authorisations from the Afghan government that would afford them more latitude with other programmes as quickly as possible. After the first round of negotiations, expectations ran high among the leaders of the armed opposition for the opening of new projects in the regions under their control. While seeking to consolidate its existing programmes, MSF thus undertook, as early as the spring of 2010, to assess new areas for interventions, hoping they could be set up in independent facilities. The two provinces chosen for this second operational phase were Khost and Kunduz.

The heartland of the Haqqani network in southeast Afghanistan, Khost was also the location of the main OEF (Operation Enduring Freedom) base in the country from where counter-terrorism operations across the border with Pakistan were carried out. Suspicions were therefore running high when the MSF team met with the elders of the local tribes, but the organisation's Haqqani contacts and the unique asset it had to offer helped to build confidence. In line with the available health data, the elders expressed a need for mother and child healthcare. MSF could set up a programme involving female expatriates, which, as the elders had to acknowledge, was the only way to ensure that local women would be cared for. Emboldened by this perspective, one of the elders suggested including mental health in the programme to address what he saw as a worrying trend of suicides among women in the region. For an expatriate team to be able to settle in the town of Khost and launch such a programme, MSF first had to undertake a new round of negotiations to obtain security guarantees from all the warring parties.

Access to the city of Kunduz was less of a security issue, but the situation in the districts was a different matter altogether. Kunduz had been the first northern province where the IEA had expanded its influence and fighting had increased over the previous year. As armed confrontation was a relatively recent phenomenon, the local health system had not yet experienced the same disruption seen in the southern provinces such as Helmand. But Kunduz had become a strategic location; a new supply route for international forces crossing the province from Tajikistan and a recent arrival of American troops under OEF command were creating widespread anticipation of an upcoming escalation in the conflict.

MSF's assessment therefore concluded that a medical presence should be negotiated as soon as possible, so as to be able to provide a timely and appropriate response to the consequences of the expected increase in violence. An expatriate team was positioned in the town of Kunduz to initiate discussions with the many local armed groups upon whom access to the districts was dependent. It was later decided to set up a trauma centre in the provincial capital to cater to the direct victims of the conflict. The project was to be housed in a private building to ensure full independence. In December 2010, the Kunduz authorities approved the project. But the war had flared up more quickly than anticipated with fighting and suicide bombings killing many of MSF's contacts in government and the opposition alike. This further complicated negotiations, and still the conditions for the organisation to start its project had not been met. In particular, without agreement on a referral system allowing wounded patients to be taken in safety from the districts to the MSF facility without risk of arrest or attack, not all the parties would be able to benefit from the project.

Negotiations regarding MSF's intervention in the provinces of Khost and Kunduz are still ongoing in the spring of 2011, at a time when domestic and international pressure on the Karzai government, the increasing stakes in the political negotiations between the belligerents and the Obama administration's commitment to begin withdrawing US troops in the summer, are all bringing about rapid changes in the political and military environment in Afghanistan. In this context, expectations weighing on MSF remain high. As a representative of the IEA bluntly put it: "We cannot guarantee your safety if you don't produce some real work".

When the two MSF members conducting an assessment mission in July 2007 met with various departments of the Karzai government, they noted that for all the expressions of welcome they received, there was a degree of ambivalence regarding the possibility of the medical agency coming back to Afghanistan: "MSF represents the past, the war and in different ministries there are also concerns and misunderstanding [...]. [Some officials] make clearly the link between our return and a deterioration of the situation in the South".[24] Again, in December 2010, as the Kunduz provincial authorities were about to sign the agreement authorising MSF to start its war-wounded programme, an official remarked in essence that he saw MSF's return to the province as both a good sign and a bad sign.

These remarks point to the same evidence, namely that humanitarian action is a symptom of war, not a cure—of war, at least. They also highlight what this chapter has attempted to show: for MSF's action to be accepted, the main political and military stakeholders in the war have to recognise the conflict as such and to have an interest in the medical services the agency can deliver. The situation prevailing in Afghanistan today is no less polarised than it was when MSF left the country in 2004 and it is no doubt far more violent. The key change from the perspective of the humanitarian actor is that medical operations in conflict-ridden areas are now seen by the competing warring-parties as building, to varying degrees, their own claim for legitimacy.

MSF has been able so far to play along with these evolving perceptions by demonstrating that its medical assistance could appeal to each side. It remains no doubt a fragile equation, which to date has allowed little improvement in access to the population trapped in war-affected rural areas. To be sure, the current scaling-up phase does contribute to a higher standing for MSF in the eyes of its high level interlocutors, but for this to last, continuity in interactions and perceived interests is crucial. This in turn depends not only on MSF's negotiating skills but even more so on the dynamics of the war—or of a violent peace. Therefore, rather than trying to gauge the size of the "humanitarian space" in Afghanistan, it may well be more accurate to consider the passing opportunities and risks of this humanitarian moment.

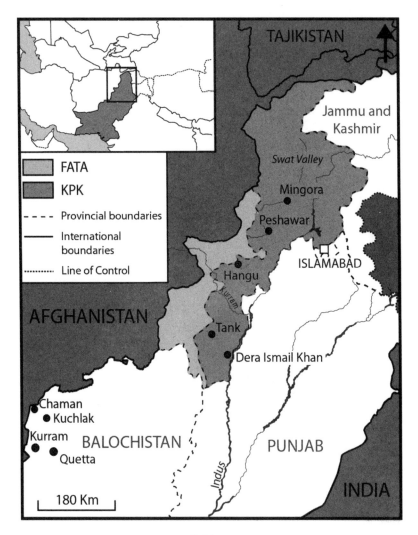

Pakistan

PAKISTAN

THE OTHER SIDE OF THE COIN

Jonathan Whittall

Between 2008 and 2010, internal conflicts and the so-called "global war on terror" in the northwest regions of Pakistan led to the displacement of 4.2 million people.[1] Since 2007, the people in the Federally Administered Tribal Areas (FATA) and Khyber Pakhtunkhwa Province (KPK)[2] have been living with the threat of fighting between the Pakistani army and armed opposition groups such as Tehrik-el-Taliban Pakistan (TTP), US drone attacks and sectarian violence. The Afghan Taliban now use the FATA region that borders Afghanistan as a launching pad for its operations against the Coalition forces. The TTP also uses the FATA as a base for its attacks against the Pakistani state. Given its very limited access to the tribal areas, MSF knows little about the population's medical needs. Most of MSF's programmes are confined to the province of KPK, close to the FATA, where the army allows the organisation to address the inadequacies in hospital services. However, the need for medical assistance is in all probability even more vital in the FATA where health workers are often unwilling to work due to the lack of security. MSF's position in Pakistan has been largely based on its principles of independence, neutrality and impartiality—which have been implemented through its decision not to accept any funding from governments for its operations in the region. The organisation has made every effort to distinguish itself from the counter-insurgency humanitarianism promoted by the authorities. But how successful have these efforts been in securing access to the most vulnerable populations?

In northwestern Pakistan, the army and international donors accord humanitarian aid a pivotal role in their "stabilisation" strategy intended to establish the government's legitimacy. In practice, counter-insurgency (COIN) priorities determine where national and international aid is delivered and who receives it. The army denies humanitarian organisations access to regions where it is conducting counter-insurgency operations until such a time as the area is pronounced "cleared" and ready for "reconstruction". This is the case for all of the FATA as it was for the districts of Dera Ismael Khan and Tank in KPK in 2010, where displaced people had gathered. In 2009 and 2010, MSF made an attempt in vain to support the health facilities in Dera Ismael Khan. Even after the floods of 2010, these areas remained off limits to MSF despite the increase in need for healthcare assistance. The official explanation given to MSF by the army was its inability to ensure the safety of international staff. But as of 2009, the army has prohibited all discussion between MSF and the TTP, even if only to negotiate guarantees of security that it couldn't deliver itself.

Although the army responded to the food, shelter and healthcare needs of the people displaced by its military operations, there was a significant lack in the delivery of assistance, particularly to those communities considered as having links to "terrorists". A collective punishment enshrined in the Frontier Crimes Regulation Act (FCR) results in aid being distributed according to region of origin rather than need. Areas that people have fled from have to be "notified" as "affected" before a person can be considered for assistance. Khyber Agency in the FATA is an example; never having been officially recognised as "affected" by conflict, the internally displaced people (IDPs) there have received almost no assistance.

This manipulation of aid has been largely supported by the United States and the United Nations, which, in effect, endorse Pakistan's stabilisation policy. As illustrated by the UN's 2010 Humanitarian Response Plan, which was introduced by a letter from the Pakistani government explaining its counter-insurgency activities in Khyber-Pakhtunkhwa/FATA, the UN and even its specialised agencies such as the HCR and WFP are clearly supporting one of the parties to the conflict. In addition, US funding is allocated according to objectives of "stabilisation through development" to which the "capacity building" actions of many NGOs contribute—often to the detriment of the capacity for emergency response.

According to one IDP interviewed in March 2010, "America is paying the people who are fighting against us and destroying our homes [referring to the Pakistani army] and then they are giving the relief. We don't trust that".[3] Based on MSF's experience in the region, such suspicion is widespread and has consequences on the ability of the broader NGO community to respond. Aware of the mistrust of the armed opposition groups and part of the population due to NGO links to US funding and the UN, many NGOs often restrict their interventions to areas where they don't run the risk of becoming targets.

In this context, MSF tried to move way from a role of assisting the counter-insurgency and stabilisation strategy in the region by extending its programmes to "non-cleared" areas and "terrorist populations". The main challenge was to gain the acceptance of all the different political and military agents—those who either supported or opposed the government. This tension was well illustrated by MSF's response to the healthcare situation in Swat.

MSF and US-Supported Stabilisation in Swat

MSF first worked in the Swat valley in KPK province in 2008 to 2009 when the armed opposition groups were in control of the area. Pakistani nationals ran operations with the support of international staff who made occasional visits. In order to be authorised to work in the valley, the Pakistani authorities demanded that MSF obtain security clearance from the opposition. The organisation had direct access to the opposition high command who themselves maintained dialogue with the state at that time. MSFs strategic partnership with the Swat Doctors Society, the supply of medicines and equipment for emergency rooms, and the setting up of an ambulance service enhanced the reputation of the organisation as a recognised medical service provider. MSF accepted to intervene without the presence of any international staff, as the parties involved in the conflict did not want to be responsible for the security of expatriates. This compromise was made because it was possible to talk to the opposition. Following a series of security incidents, which included the murder of two MSF staff in a clearly marked ambulance, MSF was forced to close its projects in the district in May 2009.

Between May and July 2009, the Pakistani army launched a major offensive in the Swat valley which caused the displacement of over three million people and led to the opposition losing control over the region. By 2010, the centre of the conflict was confined to the FATA where MSF had no access, apart from a small project in the Kurram district. MSF returned to Swat in May 2010 to re-open the emergency room at Mingora district hospital after the offensive had been proclaimed a success by the Pakistani government and the area proclaimed "cleared" and accorded priority status for "development for stabilisation".

The government of Pakistan outlined its stabilisation strategy for Swat in the "Malakand comprehensive stabilisation and socio-economic development plan".[4] In the section on "delivery of basic social services", there is specific reference to the need to restore, expand and upgrade health infrastructure. In addition to this infrastructure funding, the US government provided approximately 36 million dollars of direct aid to the KPK government, with 12 million dollars earmarked for Recovery, Staffing and Supplies for the Department of Health.[5] Where there are funds, there are NGOs. In the case of Swat, it is estimated that up to eighty national and international NGOs arrived in the Swat valley after the military offensive.

MSF's decision to return to Swat after the offensive was based not on a desire to rebuild the area in support of a stabilisation agenda, but on medical needs. The Mingora hospital emergency room was barely functioning and, despite claims that the conflict was over, insecurity remained, as witnessed by the sporadic influx of numerous wounded patients. The principal challenge faced by the organisation was how to function in these conditions without compromising its ability to be accepted by local groups opposed to the government and its COIN strategy in and around Swat. This was particularly important as the authorities made clear to MSF that they would not tolerate MSF treating "militants" in its health facility.

As a preventive measure, MSF, bolstered by the trust of the population gained during its previous intervention in the region, decided to make a public statement as part of a broader strategy to engage with the population in Swat. A press release in the local media explained what its intentions were in returning to the area. "MSF is coming back to Swat to address very specific medical needs that we have identified at Mingora hospital. As an emergency medical organisation that is focused solely on providing lifesaving care, MSF is not involved in rebuilding Swat after the offensive, nor are we part of any military or political strategy. For our activities in Pakistan, we do not accept any government funding, choosing only to rely on private funds from individuals".[6] MSF also decided to no longer refer to itself in its contacts with different parties as an NGO—synonymous with US funding, connections to the UN and faith-based organisations—but rather as a private medical organisation and, later, as a medical humanitarian association. It was also necessary to find the right partners to implement its programmes. This required extensive networking with various groups within the community, in Swat and in the region. Specifically, MSF tried to establish relationships with madrasas (religious schools) and national NGOs, who played an important role in the response to the displacement caused by the conflict and the floods in 2010. The fact that MSF engaged with organisations considered by the west as the competition in the scramble for the population's "hearts and minds", was both a vital step in realigning people's perception of the organisation and ensuring its programmes reached those most in need.

In the other areas of northwest Pakistan where MSF had been unable to negotiate access after 2009, the organisation might have been able to operate, had it agreed to work through national NGOs or with Pakistani nationals exclusively. This is how MSF managed to set up its project in the district of Kurram Agency in the FATA, as it had in Swat in 2008. This would have allowed MSF to access places such as Dera Ismail Khan and parts of the FATA. Yet the decision was taken in 2010 not to replicate this strategy in other parts of the FATA and KPK: in such a highly political and contested context, and without direct dialogue with the opposition, MSF considered it essential to have mixed national and international teams, because international staff can provide a buffer between national staff and community pressures, including pressures from armed groups. This was a lesson learnt from Swat where the MSF national staff running the projects were put under immense pressure to take increased security risks to respond to the needs of their community, resulting in the loss of two MSF ambulance staff in 2009.

The organisation's international staff would have been allowed access if it had decided to resort to Pakistani army escorts. But, as these would have been provided by one of the parties to the conflict, they would have made MSF a target.

Navigating Dangerous Waters

In a context such as Pakistan, MSF's ability to increase its safe operating environment, at least in the eyes of the armed opposition, is less about how its principles are understood and more about how its politics are perceived. The affirmation of "neutrality and independence" that MSF lobbies for so vigorously in Pakistan is so against the practices of state-led humanitarianism at the service of counter-insurgency and stabilisation that it becomes a political position in itself that can lead to a degree of acceptance. Because humanitarian organisations in Pakistan embrace western political priorities, the opposition accords a certain value to MSF's distinct position.

MSF is still only able to operate in those areas to which the government allows it access. Ultimately, MSF's ability to navigate in the COIN context should be judged in the light of its actual capacity to conduct its activities for those who are denied assistance. MSF's access to parts of KPK such as Hangu and Timergara, particularly by its international staff, represents a significant achievement. The extent of its operations in these areas is far greater than any other humanitarian organisation has achieved. However, despite these successes, MSF has been unable to gain enough leverage to access FATA, where needs are likely to be most acute, with compromises that the organisation deems acceptable.

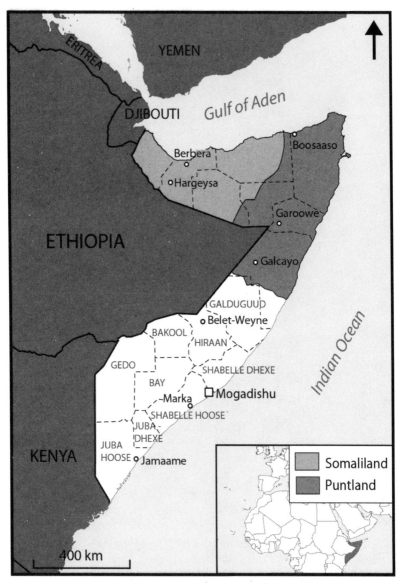

YEMEN

Gulf of Aden

ERITREA

DJIBOUTI

ETHIOPIA

Berbera

oHargeysa

oBoosaaso

Garoowe

oGalcayo

GALDUGUUD

oBelet-Weyne

BAKOOL

HIRAAN

GEDO

BAY

SHABELLE DHEXE

Marka

☐Mogadishu

SHABELLE HOOSE

JUBA DHEXE

JUBA HOOSE

oJamaame

KENYA

Indian Ocean

400 km

Somaliland

Puntland

Somalia

SOMALIA
EVERYTHING IS OPEN TO NEGOTIATION

Michaël Neuman (interview with Benoît Leduc)

This chapter is the result of conversations held from June to December 2010 between Michaël Neuman, director of studies at CRASH—MSF and Benoît Leduc, head of mission and then operations manager for Somalia for the French section of Médecins Sans Frontières from December 2006 to September 2010. As a result, the positions of the Belgian, Spanish, Dutch and Swiss sections also operating in Somalia are not covered in any detail.

Introduction

Médecins Sans Frontières, which had provided assistance to Somali-Ethiopian refugees in Somalia since 1979, quickly came to see the risks and challenges of working in the country. In January 1987, ten members of a team in Tuj Walaje in the north were kidnapped by Somali-land separatists and, in April 1988, the Dutch section of MSF was working in Hargeisa when the town was hit by a heavy bombing raid. The decade that followed began with a conflict that was the outcome of a process initiated years earlier and combined the collapse of the government with an explosion in the number of private armies built around individuals, clans and entrepreneurs.[1] Following the fall of President Siad Barre in 1991, MSF embarked on a series of operations in a Mogadishu torn apart by clan rivalry, in rural areas with displaced people and in Kenya among the Somali refugees who had fled the war. One of MSF's main concerns was to limit the consequences of the famine which, from spring 1992 onwards, was to trigger one of the first international "military-humanitarian" interventions of the post-Cold War period. Relief operations were carried out in one of the most dangerous environments MSF had ever encountered. The intensity of the fighting as well as the direct threats made against MSF's employees led to a number of personnel evacuations.

From April 1992 to March 1995, the United Nations ran several consecutive missions intended to ensure compliance with a ceasefire by the main warring factions, as well as the safety of humanitarian aid. Successive reinforcements of the international force, however, were to contribute to its becoming directly involved in the conflict. Civilian and military losses increased, while the international forces themselves perpetrated war crimes. The confusion between humanitarian aid and international military intervention reached a climax. Not wanting to be further associated with violence perpetrated in the name of humanitarianism and facing growing security threats and the Somali population's hostility towards foreigners, the French section of MSF decided to withdraw from the country in May 1993. This decision was also based on the decline in mortality caused by the famine. Over the years that followed the country remained a focus of confrontation between political-military leaders.[2] In spite of regular interruptions, MSF continued to work on projects to provide assistance to the Somali population. In 1997 expatriate doctor Ricardo Marques was assassinated in the hospital in Baidoa supported by the French section, which had returned to the country two years earlier. This incident prompted a second withdrawal.

A letup in the fighting in Mogadishu nine years later enabled MSF-France to return to Somalia. During the summer of 2006, the Islamic Courts Union (ICU), established in the mid-1990s in an attempt to restore order in Mogadishu, took control of the capital, which they intended to use as a testing ground for an Islamic Somalia. The population of Mogadishu saw a period of calm it had not known for fifteen years and the international airport, closed since 1995, reopened. A window of opportunity emerged for relief organisations that hoped security conditions were about to improve. The opportunity turned out to be short-lived. In December 2006, the Ethiopian government, fearing the establishment of a radical Islamist regime on its doorstep, launched a large-scale offensive against the ICU and defeated it.

The conflict escalated with renewed vigour, exacerbated by its internationalisation against the backdrop of the "global war on terror", and opposed transnational Jihadist networks to western powers, the United Nations (UN) and their regional allies. The rebel movement became increasingly radicalised, which resulted in a series of breakaway groups. One of them, Al Shabaab, initially an ICU "youth movement", became an independent organisation with a small number of highly radicalised individuals. The troops confronted the Transitional Federal Government (TFG), supported by the UN and the AMISOM, an African Union mission created in 2007. Yet the TFG, divided and powerless, was never able to control more than a few districts of Mogadishu.

It is in this context that the French section of MSF did its utmost to find a way to provide assistance in the country. The organisation was forced in a series of never-ending negotiations to compromise in a number of areas: the security of its personnel, the recourse to armed guards, the choice of its action, the standard of its relief operations, its contribution to the war efforts of the warring parties, as well as its ability to speak out.

Discussion

> For many at MSF in Paris, the situation in Somalia could be summed up in a few words: clans, the memory of the death of Ricardo Marques, and complexity. It was the embodiment of operating in unacceptable security conditions and dependence on armed groups. The French section, which had withdrawn from the country in 1997, examined the possibility of a return in 2006. What was the background to the debate?

In the wake of their victory over the Alliance for the Restoration of Peace and Counter-Terrorism (ARPCT)[3] in June 2006, the ICU took control of Mogadishu. The residents of the city who were, in appearance at least, completely unarmed, returned to a level of security they had not enjoyed for fifteen years. The change in circumstances afforded those who supported a return of MSF's French section to Somalia the opportunity to float the idea once again. An exploratory mission was carried out in the summer of 2006 in Mogadishu and in the port city of Merka in the south of the country, to establish contacts and assess the reality of the situation on the ground. The return to war following the Ethiopian army's intervention in Somalia at the end of 2006 encouraged this approach. It was then that I was charged with monitoring the situation and looking at potential projects for the country.

There were numerous discussions at MSF on whether we should start up a new project. The director of operations was opposed to the use of armed guards, and brought up the question of the potential security risks for our teams in re-launching activities in Somalia. In addition, four sections of MSF were already working in the country, and that gave some people sufficient grounds to argue that there was no need for the French section to be there.

> Let's go back to the issue of armed guards. In Afghanistan, in Eritrea and on many occasions in other situations, the organisation has used combatants to ensure the safety of its teams and convoys. Whilst humanitarian aid should not be imposed by force, the use of armed escorts has sometimes been seen in the history of the organisation as a condition for providing assistance. What were the arguments in the debate that prompted MSF to resort to armed guards in carrying out its operations in Somalia?

During the discussions that preceded the decision to resume operations, the reasons put forward to oppose the use of armed guards were based on MSF's experience in Somalia and in other countries: the risk of getting involved in funding the conflict, putting the teams in greater danger and becoming dependent on the militias sometimes added to the issue of the neutrality of operations. In the early 1990s, the use of militias was a prerequisite for taking action, from which it then became impossible to extricate ourselves. Although they were supposed to defend the organisation, they would themselves create incidents to generate a further reinforcing of the system. From the mid-1990s onwards, the teams began to reduce the number of guards and to limit our contractual relationships with the militias: MSF, if only to a small degree, was potentially able to play a part in creating the conditions for violence. Using guards meant that we ran the risk of a member of MSF staff killing someone. The numerous security incidents we had faced in the past meant this was a legitimate argument.

But in Somalia, armed guards were above all a necessity, not a choice. On our first visits to the country, we also said we didn't want armed guards. And then we realised that even the smallest of shops had a guard armed with a Kalashnikov. Since the 1990s, security in Somalia had been completely privatised. It was simply something that was accepted by the MSF teams working at the time and that we came to acknowledge. All Somali hospitals are equipped with a kind of cloakroom where owners check in their weapons in exchange for a number. That's just the way it is. So, after talking it through, that was the reality MSF decided to accept.

> What were the stages involved in re-launching operations?

One of the members of the exploratory mission in summer 2006 had been the head of mission in 1997, and he met his former deputy at the hotel in Mogadishu. Like many other Somalis, the latter had come to see what was happening in the city with a view to starting up activities again. He was based in Kismayo, in the south of Somalia, and helped us with a visit to Jamaame, a town in the region. A rural area that had for the most part been spared from the fighting, it had a landing strip. This was vital as travelling by car quickly became too dangerous.

Then, of course, there were clearly identified medical needs, as is the case in all Somali rural areas and, above all, the fact that there was no one to provide care. We carried out a few exploratory missions in the surrounding villages. There were heavy floods between November 2006 and January 2007. According to what we were told, children died of diarrhoea because of a shortage of drinking water—the people drank water from the river. Aware of the impact of the floods on the harvest, we feared that the nutritional situation would deteriorate too.

There were many discussions over whether it was appropriate to intervene in Jamaame. Many people felt that the process would slow down our objective of starting up in Mogadishu, which was seen as a priority insofar as the capital was heavily populated and the focus of the conflict. In fact, the project in Jamaame started up very quickly. Some people in the region were already familiar with MSF through our work in Kismayo in the 1990s. The village representatives quickly appointed a single point of contact to manage the vehicles, recruit unskilled staff and rent buildings. We explained and emphasised the principles that underpin MSF operations, namely neutrality in relation to the conflict, our independence from the political authorities and the imperative of being able to provide care for everyone. We had a team in place as of March 2007. In April, we turned our attention back to starting the project in Mogadishu.

I think the work we did in Jamaame was invaluable. It's important to remember that we had started working in Somalia on the basis of a few previous experiences. It was as if we were paralysed, we understood nothing—or maybe we only understood the risks. In Jamaame we were able to learn again how to operate in Somalia in the right conditions: how to travel around, how to carry out swift nutritional assessments, and how to talk to our contacts to gain an understanding of the health situation.

There was only one clan, which had a reputation for keeping out of the conflict, and the people were asking for help. This enabled us to understand the role of the elders in the village and that of the chiefs who represent each of the clan's seven sub-clans, and to tackle the question of sorting out cars, houses and armed guards, all issues we would face in Mogadishu. Hiring a car in Somalia results in a series of compromises. You have to forget what you learned as a logistician; that a car should drive straight, brake and have safety belts. There, it's first and foremost about finding out who owns it, what the power relationships are between clans and individuals and evaluating the risks of reprisals against the teams. We would never have been able to figure all that out in Mogadishu, what with the war, population displacements, the multitude of clans, and so on.

Besides, there was an advantage in having a rural base and a project with seemingly more long-term viability in terms of security. So, until 2008, there were almost no team evacuations. Some of the reasons behind starting up the project in Jamaame were institutional. We didn't know how long it would take to set up a project in Mogadishu, so it was also a way of getting off the ground and a justification for setting up a team in Nairobi to support Mogadishu.

As far as armed guards were concerned, we discussed different options in order to rid ourselves of some of the constraints they engender. MSF's guards are not under contract and we do not manage them directly; we give the people's representatives a sum of money and they decide and run the organisational aspects. But the questions remain. What instructions should we give the guards? How do we manage their relationship with us?

> The team that carried out the first exploratory mission in Mogadishu during the summer of 2006 had proposed working on maternity and obstetric care, but this was rejected. There weren't sufficient indicators and the risks the teams would be taking seemed too high. The fall of the Islamic courts and the return to fighting in early 2007 prompted a fresh round of discussions. In the end, it was agreed to make surgery the focus of the project. Why not reconcile both priorities? How did the launch of the project in Mogadishu go?

We were faced with the difficulty of obtaining reliable indicators right from our very first visits to Somalia. There is no official data and the numbers can be rigged because they can't be verified. MSF, with its culture of working with numbers and used to dealing with epidemiological tools, finds it difficult to go ahead with a project based merely on the teams' gut feelings or intuition. How to grasp the concept of need, when the whole situation feels like an emergency: population displacements, recurring nutritional crises, mediocre immunisation rates, general insecurity, etc.? It was difficult to carry out the actual assessments as the lack of public health facilities was, to some extent, compensated for by pharmacies and private surgeries. We really had no understanding of Somali healthcare practices.

In some ways it was a little simpler in Mogadishu after the Ethiopian intervention; there was a war, and people were wounded. Given the security conditions we were facing at the time, we felt it was important to act where there was risk to life. Surgery was the obvious choice. We carried out an assessment in January 2007 and another in April 2007. At the time, the Somali capital was in turmoil. Ethiopian and government troops were engaged in major offensives against the Islamist combatants in the northern districts of the city. According to the UNHCR, the fighting left over 1,000 civilian casualties and 350,000 people were displaced, primarily in the Afgooye corridor, located some thirty kilometres to the west of the capital. The Ethiopians systematically looted and destroyed the medical centres that could have provided assistance to the Islamist rebels.

Evaluation missions were carried out in various facilities in and around the city. We wanted to be based in an existing facility, to make the procedures required for launching the project and the negotiations regarding security easier. We looked at what was available. Of the 800 hospital beds available in January 2007, there were only 250 left by June. The only surgery facilities were those supported by the ICRC.

But they were not fully accessible to the opposition forces, partly because of their location.

The hospital in the suburban district of Daynile in the northwest of the city was thought to be a potentially good location. It had received an influx of patients and was struggling, but it was in good condition. Located right in the middle of a displaced persons' camp, it was some way from the centre. This was crucial, because a facility in the centre of the city would have put us right in the firing line and people would have found it hard to reach.

But warlord and local entrepreneur Mohamed Qanyare, a key figure in Mogadishu, already controlled the hospital. Our relationship with Qanyare was the subject of some profound disagreements with other sections of MSF, which saw it as a risk for the security of our projects. First close to the TFG, he had moved away and then joined again. He had been bankrolled by the United States, notably within the framework of the 2006 Alliance for the Restoration of Peace and Counter-Terrorism (ARPCT).

We explained to Mohamed Qanyare the importance of providing access for everyone. He seemed to accept this and withdrew from the management of the hospital. He said: "I'll deal with security in the area. As far as the rest goes, talk to so-and-so, and so-and-so, and so-and-so".

Qanyare is a Murusade chief, a sub-clan of the Hawiye clan. There were Murusades more or less everywhere, both among Al Shabaab and within President Yusuf's government and the National Security Agency, which is responsible for intelligence and counter-terrorism. These multiple allegiances, of course, result in a highly complex situation, but we can also put them to our advantage to create opportunities for discussions with the various players involved.

We were able fairly quickly to secure guarantees that combatants from all factions would be able to receive care at the hospital. Everyone agreed to play the game, albeit reluctantly. To some extent, Qanyare took a gamble on his reputation in the operation. He had stood in the 2004 presidential elections and was still counting on carving out a political career for himself, and wanted to show that he was open to all the clans. I think he both played this role and acted as a gatekeeper, opening the door to foreigners and thereby making an agreement with the clan possible.

From the rebels' point of view, it was in their interest to support assistance for their wounded and displaced populations and to encourage the aid organisations to attest to the crimes committed by the Ethiopian army with the support of the government militias. They knew that we were going to work with someone who they had been at war with, while Mohammed Qanyare knew that he was giving us access to a hospital that would be used to provide care for enemy combatants.

> Taking into account the interests of the parties to the conflict raises questions over how operational decisions are made, demonstrating that they are not purely the result of MSF's assessment of the needs of the population.

The decisions were based on a combination of different criteria. There were discussions on whether we should gear our operations towards paediatrics or surgery. Paediatrics would have met some real needs and would have been easier to put in place as the technical requirements would have been less complex. But we started with surgery—for which there was also an overwhelming need—because it was what the key players and leading figures we were able to meet asked us to do. If we had opened a nutrition or paediatric centre, the rebels, the radical Islamist militias, the Murusades and all the other groups would have been less tolerant in their attitude towards the project. It is likely the hospital would have been looted at some point or another.

During our visit in April 2007, at the same time as the discussions on starting up our project in Mogadishu, we were put in contact with a group of doctors who were close to the rebel movement. They were operating in secret and described the violent actions of the Ethiopian army against medical facilities. They stressed the importance of a neutral facility able to treat the wounded, regardless of who they are. We talked to them about our project in Daynile and working with Qanyare. Although they were reluctant, they understood that rebel combatants would have access to the hospital. To support them in their medical intervention, we donated medical equipment, a radiology device and operating tables worth over 120,000 euros. Opposition doctors no longer had the resources to care for the population and wanted treatment facilities to re-open. The donations gave us the opportunity to meet their needs and build relationships with the doctors; it was also a way for us to pay the price of our relationship with Qanyare while negotiating the setting up of a project in Daynile. We had no direct control over what use they would make of the equipment. But we decided to go ahead in spite of the fears of other MSF sections, who maintained that this so-called support for the Islamist opposition could jeopardise all our projects in the country.

We also implemented water supply projects in the displaced persons' camps established around the hospital after the wave of displacements during spring 2007 and distributed jerry cans of water and blankets. Supporting the local people was a way of protecting the hospital.

> While setting up the project, MSF was keen to formalise the sharing of resources with its various key players. What were the strategies adopted?

Our ability to set up and maintain the project relied primarily on establishing a body to govern the hospital, namely a sort of Board of Directors independent of MSF. We continue to provide "indirect" management, avoiding as far as possible any involvement in personal, political and local clan disputes. We do not select the dozen or so members of the Board, who are co-opted. Usually leading figures in the district, they are frequently relatives and friends of Qanyare and the Murusades.

If there's a problem, we say to them: "You're the Board, it's your hospital, you manage it and we'll support it". When we wanted to pull out of supplying water by lorry to drill instead, we discussed it with the Board. It was the Board that negotiated access to the land and then sorted out terminating the lorry rentals. We find these negotiations unfathomable, and do not get involved. All we do is convey messages: "If MSF is threatened, we might have to cut short the projects".

As far as recruitment is concerned, we decided to take a gamble: if we focused on skills, we would find the diversity of clans vital to reach our patients. We recruit using written tests and questionnaires supervised by international staff. We have promoted the transparency of the system in conjunction with the Board. If everyone is entitled to take part and staff are recruited for their skills rather than their clan, people are ready to go along with it. In April 2008, we organised a test to recruit twenty nurses which was taken by 535 people.

As in Jamaame, security is arranged at arm's length. The budget allocated to armed guards is included in a package we give to the hospital designed to fund its running costs, including non-surgical medical activities in which we have no direct involvement.

> Since the project began, over 12,000 patients have been treated in the hospital, with over 50% of injuries caused by the war. That said, the situation has changed hugely. The region is now controlled by

Al Shabaab and Qanyare's influence has decreased. Given this context, can civilian populations and combatants from different factions still access the hospital?

During the first months of the project, patients came primarily from areas in the immediate vicinity of the hospital. There was a significant proportion of women and children among the injured who had been victims of the bombing raids: over 56% between October and December 2007, and over 53% in 2008. Gradually, patients started to come from a wider area and we were reassured that the whole of the population, whatever their clan, had access to the hospital. We are now effectively in a neighbourhood controlled by the Islamist opposition, with the war-wounded coming from this area. This is less the case for patients not wounded in the war and who come from a much more diverse range of geographical areas.

It's highly likely that some armed factions refuse to go to the hospital, but that is certainly not the case for women and children. It's difficult to be sure. They have fallen as a proportion of all those treated for war-related injuries since 2008, but the figures vary as the conflict evolves along with the nature and location of the fighting. As soon as there are bombing raids in residential areas, the proportion increases again. Conversely, during periods of intense and direct clashes such as we have seen since the beginning of the year, more of our admissions are combatants. But we must continue to closely monitor this issue of access without distinction to the hospital.

In these conditions, we are sometimes seen by some political players, the African Union mission officers, for example, as the opposition's war surgeons. This is when we need to remind people of the fundamentals of providing access to medical facilities in times of war, namely that injured and unarmed combatants are classed as non-combatants. What's more, they only represent a proportion of our patients. We can also remind people of our support for the medical department of the hospital, where 70% of in-patients are women and children.

In Jamaame too we have had to deal with a change in authority and the fact that Al Shabaab has taken power. At the beginning of our intervention, the elders were in power and in charge of the judicial system, the police, the prison and the market—even if a representative of the TFG was present. When Al Shabaab regained control of the town in May 2008, the elders were removed from power and in some cases accused of corruption. They have now been partially reintegrated into the community, because Al Shabaab has probably understood the advantages of having their support in administering the region.

> In January 2008, an attack on a team from the Dutch section of MSF in Kismayo caused the death of three employees, a Somali, a Kenyan and a Frenchman. These murders and an ongoing deterioration in the country's security situation instigated a major review of MSF's operating methods. All projects switched to what is known as "remote management", which means that day-to-day project management is carried out by national staff working remotely with international staff. It is, to some extent, comparable to the armed guards' issue; it shatters the idealised vision of the giving of aid. Is humanitarian aid not fundamentally about our relationship with other people: the doctor from here who goes to care for people there? The arguments opposed to this method of management raise questions about the neutrality and independence of national staff, as well as the issue of control of resources. How do we resolve these dilemmas?

The attack in Kismayo in January 2008 led to the withdrawal of international staff from all MSF projects but, after a few weeks of internal discussions, we sent teams back to Jamaame and Daynile. The assassination of Al Shabaab leader Aden Hashi Ayro[4] by the United States in May 2008 created a power vacuum that a number of Jihadist factions were able to take advantage of and which drove some of them to become more radical, more quickly. This fragmentation of the Islamist rebellion had a very high cost in terms of humanitarian workers' security. At the same time, we saw an escalation in the rejection of humanitarian aid—seen purely and simply as providing support to the Islamists—by many supporters of the TFG. Until Sheikh Sharif Sheikh Ahmed was elected head of the government in January 2009, attacks on humanitarian workers by TFG fighters were no less dangerous than those carried out by Al Shabaab.[5]

In the period that preceded Ayro's death, we had been able to maintain contact with the opposition via the Murusade and medical networks, and established a constructive working relationship with Al Shabaab. The organisation even wrote to us in January 2008 to offer us their encouragement. But as soon as non-Murusade Islamist rebels arrived in Daynile, it became more difficult for us to negotiate visits, particularly as the journey between the airport and the hospital became even more dangerous, due to the fighting and the risk of kidnap.

We were forced to restrict ourselves to organising occasional visits to Jamaame, where we had an expatriate team. In Daynile, we had started the project without any international staff present on an ongoing basis, not only because of the risks of foreigners being targeted but also the potential for collateral damage—getting caught in crossfire, attacks, etc. Our decision not to get involved in non-surgical medical activities was also due to insufficient expatriate staff. We moved from this kind of intermittent mode to making infrequent and last-minute lightning visits. The expatriate team is still based in Nairobi, so project management now relies much more heavily on Somali personnel than it did in the past. Of course some people have been able to adjust to a situation where they are paid a salary and have access to resources and drugs with less supervision. Organising visits to Daynile is an additional source of stress for staff because they have to organise and pay close attention to our security.

The future of the programme will depend on the relation between the security issue and the obligation to monitor; from their side, a member of the Board in Daynile explains that, "We know that if something goes wrong, it'll be the end of the hospital"; and from our point of view, as our head of mission explained, "If nothing happens, meaning that if we don't go there, that'll be the end of the hospital too". And that's where we are today.

Our biggest constraint is our limited ability to expand our activities and our capacity to respond to emergencies. In August 2010, the number of displaced people living in the camps in the Daynile area was probably around 110,000. There was a very high level of need and the aid provided was inadequate. A few organisations, such as the Red Crescent, do a small amount of work in the camps. In normal times, we would probably decide on a major intervention, supplying water, purification and distribution systems, providing medical care, etc. But the camps are Al Shabaab's constituency and are under its tight control. Our staff are not always comfortable with the idea of working in them. Generally speaking, the threats faced by the local employees are immense and the risk to their safety huge and incessant.

As for checking that the resources provided by MSF are properly used, we look at as much medical, logistical and financial information as we can and, up to a certain point, all the elements of a normal project are there. We have to examine supervision, the quality of medical care and monitoring. We analyse the quantities of drugs used, activity reports and the number of registered patients. We then examine the consumption of certain sensitive and expensive drugs, as well as the reasons for and data on admissions and discharge in nutritional activities. There's some information we're not able to get hold of, such as the number of children in the nutrition programme, for example, and we do have some fictitious patients. But we encounter the same challenges in projects where expatriates are involved. Our visits to Daynile—and we haven't been back since April 2009—are, in fact, relatively ineffective. We spend our time dealing with the unplanned events that crop up on a day-to-day basis while the medical side, such as carrying out an inventory of the pharmacy, monitoring a patient, checking the quality of care and prescriptions, is reduced to a bare minimum.

This is an ongoing situation and the quality of care provided by MSF gives cause for concern. Our standards of care in Daynile are not those of our programmes in Haiti, for example. It is even hard sometimes to check our doctors' qualifications. Because of this and despite our discussions with the staff and the training we have put in place, fracture repairs and infection control are not carried out in conditions as satisfactory as we would like.

As long as the security situation continues to remain this problematic, we are unlikely to see a return to a regular expatriate presence in the near future. What's more, new constraints may well be on the horizon, notably Al Shabaab's demands regarding the nationalities of the expatriates it will authorise to visit the projects.

> In January 2008, Al Shabaab proclaimed its unequivocal allegiance to the leaders of Al Qaeda. At the same time, the international intervention was operating in a context increasingly influenced by the "war on terror". What has been the impact of this polarisation on our activities?

We are seeing a new period where the parties to the conflict are attempting to co-opt aid, in a country that has seen many such attempts. In January 2010, the WFP, against a background of accusations of misappropriation and corruption, announced it was suspending its aid programme in the centre and south of the country because of the growing number of attacks on its staff. Then, in February, Al Shabaab itself prohibited food aid from the WFP on the pretext that its operations were "politically motivated" and that they were undermining the local market. In November 2009, it issued a list of eleven conditions for the continuation of international aid, including payment of a 20,000 dollar tax every six months and the dismissal of all female staff, except for those working in treatment facilities. In August 2010, Al Shabaab announced it had banned NGOs such as World Vision, ADRA and Diakonia, accusing them of proselytising. The group is now demanding that Somali employees working on MSF projects in the area under its control pay a tax equivalent to 5% of their salary, in addition to "registration costs" of 10,000 dollars per project. It also tries to impose taxes for using the airports. Daynile is not affected, or at least the Board has been able to block the demands, which proves how important the project is to Al Shabaab.

Each Al Shabaab demand leads to more discussions on the restrictions we are prepared to accept or that it is reasonable to accept in such a complex situation: a combination of the considerable medical needs, questions regarding our ability to manage such complicated programmes and the impasse in which international intervention and the country, now embarking on yet another peace plan, find themselves.

But, international sanctions and anti-terrorist legislation do tend to limit the ability of aid organisations to work in rebel-controlled areas. It is civilians' access to aid that is undermined. As the United Nations sends out on a daily basis ever more alarming messages on the "humanitarian situation", in 2009 American donors suspended some of their funding, fearing that they could be prosecuted for providing assistance to Al Shabaab, classified since March 2008 as a terrorist organisation by the US State Department. In March 2010, the United Nations itself adopted a resolution[6] that potentially sets up the conditions for imposing sanctions on aid organisations working in areas controlled by opposition groups. In an article published in June 2009, the United Nations' special representative in Somalia, Ahmedou Ould-Abdallah, wrote that "those who claim neutrality may also be the accomplices" of the opposition. Even if it has no immediate consequences, this process makes the need to differentiate international initiatives in the eyes of both the people and the parties to the conflict all the more vital.

However, insofar as Al Shabaab controls the majority of the country and Mogadishu in particular, all we can do is accept reality. It is crucial that we ensure that patients are not selected on the basis of their allegiance to or membership of certain groups, and that we don't choose whom we talk to—including those claiming to be from Al Qaeda.

> Violence against civilians is frequent, attacks on hospitals are not irregular and our activities are restricted by security issues. In the

public arena, however, we hear much more from the United Nations than from MSF, which doesn't appear to be saying much at all. What do we want to say? What are we not allowing ourselves to say?

Initially, our communications policy was coherent with that of our operations. Keeping a low profile was the order of the day. We didn't want to say anything at all. We were afraid of everyone. Responsibility for the attack in Kismayo against MSF-Holland has never been clearly established. We were afraid of Al Shabaab, the Ethiopians, the clans, the warlords, the government and the lack of government.

In the beginning, everyone in Daynile—the local people, the staff, the rebels and then Al Shabaab—told us, "Don't talk politics, don't get involved in politics". This was the message we were given very clearly on several occasions. Maybe the strategy has paid off, given that Al Shabaab in Jamaame has expelled all other NGOs, but not MSF.

The risk we run when we speak out in such a complex situation is huge. As a result, our current public communications are purely factual and very closely linked to our activities, such as our treatment of malnourished children and the wounded in Daynile. Fear of Al Shabaab is even greater and MSF's communications must be pragmatic, as it is now more important to distance ourselves from international efforts focused on defeating Al Shabaab and offering absolute support to a transitional government running out of steam. While we were able to publish a press release appealing to the African Union not to bomb residential neighbourhoods, we have never asked Al Shabaab not to use civilians as a human shield when its members take cover in the market in Bakaraha.

Given the immensity of the medical needs and the complexity and difficulty of meeting them, we are afraid of losing what we have managed to put in place. It seems to us essential that we set ourselves apart from other international players, by not calling for the reinforcement of AMISOM, for example. But speaking out about who is responsible for the conflict is certainly more difficult to define and accept.

Translated from French by Karen Stokes

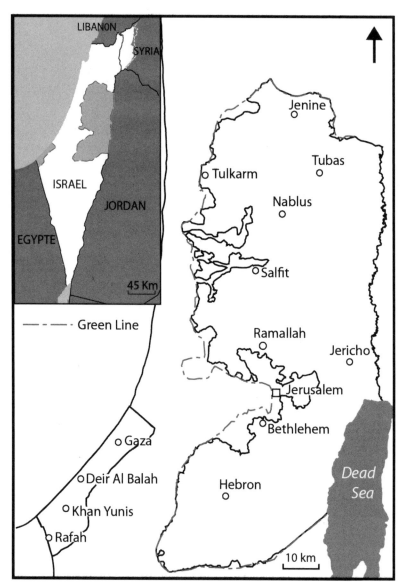

Palestinian Territories

GAZA STRIP

A PERILOUS TRANSITION

Caroline Abu-Sada

MSF began working in the Palestinian territories in 1988, a few months after the outbreak of the first Intifada. Since then, various MSF sections have attempted to attenuate the effects of Israel's occupation on Palestinians' access to certain types of healthcare. But the existence of an efficient health system has made it difficult for the organisation to find its place. For example, in Gaza in 2007, there were almost 3,800 doctors, more than 4,200 nurses and around twenty hospitals for a population of just over 1.5 million. It counted 13.6 hospitals beds per 10,000 inhabitants, against seventeen in Jordan. Furthermore, the main causes of mortality in Gaza are cardiac and cerebrovascular diseases,[1] the same as in high or intermediate income regions. MSF's projects are operating in the midst of a conflict that has been internationalised from the outset, attracting a huge amount of media attention and generating intense transnational political mobilisation. The imperative for MSF to be present in such a symbolic conflict is complicated by the difficulties in finding relevant medical programmes.

This chapter focuses on MSF's actions in the Gaza Strip between 2007 and 2010. During this period the organisation was seriously rethinking its political and operational positioning—a rethink that would call for concessions by both MSF and the government of Gaza.

The French section of MSF has been working in Gaza since 2000. Until 2005, its project was centred on psychological care, accompanied by medical-social care for people living in areas particularly hard-hit by the conflict (families whose houses had been requisitioned by the army, or were living near the settlements or in parts of the Gaza Strip where military authorisation was needed to enter or leave, etc.). After Israel's disengagement from the Gaza Strip in August 2005, MSF focused its attention on the border areas, considered to be the worst affected by the violence. Its programmes included the procurement of medicines and medical supplies for health facilities in preparation for a possible inflow of casualties. At the start of its interventions in Gaza, MSF was in contact with its usual political interlocutors: Israel, with which it negotiated visas, access to Gaza and administrative issues, and the Palestinian Authority, a nascent state body established by the 1993 Oslo Accords, based in Ramallah, in the West Bank, with which it coordinated care activities.

In January 2006, Hamas (the "Islamic Resistance Movement") won a decisive victory in the Palestinian elections. There followed a year of political tension between Fatah, the main party of the Palestinian Authority, and Hamas. In the spring of 2007, armed fighting broke out in the Gaza Strip, and in June, after a battle left more than a hundred people dead, Hamas took power. But the Palestinian Authority still had control of the West Bank, so there was now a government led by a democratically-elected party, Hamas, in the Gaza Strip, and a non-elected government led by the Fatah Party in the West Bank. The government in Gaza was immediately boycotted by part of the international community, including the United States and the European Union. Israel set up a land, air and sea blockade from which humanitarian aid was supposedly exempt. The main institutional donors made funding for non-governmental organisations dependent on an undertaking not to enter into contact with Hamas, forcing some NGOs to limit or even suspend their activities. MSF, whose projects were financed from private funds, was not affected by these constraints which, in the name of the fight against terrorism, discriminated against Palestinians unlucky enough to be living in the wrong place. In September 2007, Israel declared Gaza a "hostile entity". From that point on, Hamas was determined to demonstrate its ability to manage Gaza or, in other words, to transform itself into a ruling party. All of Hamas' strategies with the actors present, and notably MSF, were established with this one aim in mind.

In 2007, healthcare in Gaza underwent some important changes. The high number of casualties in the fighting between Palestinian factions tested the limits of its care system. In June 2007, the "Battle of Gaza" alone left more than 500 people wounded. The Palestinian hospitals coped remarkably well with the surgical requirements, but could provide little post-operative care. The climate of insecurity and the tension between the two factions also limited access to public care facilities for any patients considered to be opponents of Hamas. Furthermore, the healthcare system suffered from the rivalry between the two health ministries in Gaza and Ramallah. Fatah which ran the Palestinian Authority, ordered its health workers posted in Gaza to strike if they wanted to continue to be paid, while Hamas duplicated the administrative facilities and appointed its own health officials. The embargo—in spite of Israel's claims that medical aid would be exempt—combined with the unwillingness of the Health Ministry in Ramallah to cooperate with Gaza, made it increasingly difficult to procure medicines and medical supplies for the hospitals.

The change in context provided MSF with an opportunity to step up the medical dimension of its programmes, in addition to the psychological care it was already providing. It opened a centre offering post-operative care and physiotherapy for casualties admitted to the Palestinian hospitals in Gaza City, and set up mobile physiotherapy teams throughout the Gaza Strip. These mobile teams provided a care solution for patients whose physical incapacity kept them housebound, and for anyone whose links with Fatah prevented them from seeking treatment in Hamas-controlled health facilities. A paediatric clinic was also opened in Beit Lahiya to make up for gaps caused by the blockade and the health worker strikes. All these new activities were run out of private MSF facilities to ensure access for all patients—and because the public hospitals were already full to overflowing.

Hamas: From Indifference to a Power Struggle
and Imposed Negotiations

In a context marked by the Israeli blockade, international sanctions against Hamas and animosity between Palestinian factions, the new political situation in Gaza created problems for MSF, used to dealing only with the Palestinian Authority and the Israelis. Since arriving in the Gaza Strip in 2000, MSF had occasionally met with the leaders of Hamas, but that was before the race for the elections when it was just another opposition party. In the months following Hamas' accession to power, MSF continued to negotiate the legal conditions governing its presence in Gaza with the Palestinian Authority. The formal agreements on the provision of post-operative outpatient care and the opening of the paediatric care unit were signed in Ramallah in August 2007 and May 2008. As for the Hamas government, it initially devoted very little time to establishing formal relations with international NGOs. Its representatives, whose responsibilities were still somewhat vague as the structure of the new government was still being decided, seemed happy enough with the informal discussions they held with MSF during which they were told about the organisation's objectives and activities.

But by continuing to negotiate the legal framework of its interventions with the Palestinian Authority in Ramallah, MSF ran the risk of being seen to support Fatah in its fight against Hamas for sovereignty. Yet in September 2008, MSF called public attention to the responsibility of the political authorities, including Fatah, in the deterioration of the health situation. A press release entitled: "Gaza: politics take precedence over health", stated that: "The Palestinian Health Workers Union [pro-Fatah] is encouraging striking members to volunteer their services free of charge to patients being cared for in facilities managed by NGOs. But MSF has neither the capacity nor the legitimacy to deal with the repercussions of this crisis. Nor is it our mandate to ensure a "minimum level of service", as certain parties to this conflict have asked us to do. MSF refuses to play this role. We cannot and must not attempt to replace an entire public health system. [...] Rather than considering healthcare as an essential service, humanitarian and vital, it is being used to apply political pressure by two parties equally heedless of the consequences this could have for the population".[2] But this was the only time since Hamas had come to power in Gaza that MSF had publicly pointed the finger at the Palestinian Authority. Substituting for inadequate health systems might well be nothing new for MSF, but here it was crucial not to appear to be taking sides in the intra-Palestinian struggle, and to highlight the uncomfortable position in which all the parties to the conflict were placing it.

At the beginning of October 2008, Bernard Kouchner, France's foreign affairs minister at the time, announced after an official visit to Gaza that the French government was being provided with information by French NGOs working there. MSF immediately issued a press release, as did Médecins du Monde (MDM), refuting these unfounded and dangerous allegations which cast doubt on its intentions and jeopardised its activities. These statements by the very minister who had co-founded MSF in 1971 and MDM in 1980 only served to heighten Hamas' mistrust of foreign aid organisations.

On 27 December the Israeli army launched "Operation Cast Lead" in the Gaza Strip. The first three days of the offensive were particularly violent. As Gaza City's main hospital, Al Shifa, was struggling to cope with the massive inflow of casualties, MSF decided to increase surgical capacity by setting up a hospital in inflatable tents. The initial plan was to put these tents up in the hospital grounds, but MSF eventually set them up at the end of the offensive outside the hospital to ensure its services would be accessible to all the victims. This project was discussed with administrative staff at the Gaza Health Ministry, but the health minister himself was not informed. In January 2009, MSF signed an agreement with the Health Ministry in Ramallah to extend its post-operative activities in the Gaza Strip.

The military offensive in December 2008 and January 2009, which left 1,300 Palestinians dead, more than 5,000 injured[3] and caused large-scale material damage, marked a political turning point in Gaza. In the eyes of the population, Hamas emerged victorious. The Palestinian Authority, on the other hand, was seriously weakened, in particular due to statements made by its president, Mahmoud Abbas, on the first day of the conflict, in which he blamed Hamas for Israel's attack on Gaza. At the end of the offensive, as a number of its leaders had been killed in the fighting, Hamas reorganised its administration. These changes led to the start of a new phase in relations between MSF and the Gaza government, which soon turned into a power struggle.

Following a visit to the tent hospital in mid-July 2009 by inspectors from the Gaza Health Ministry, the minister decided to close the facility down with immediate effect on the grounds that MSF did not have the necessary authorisations and that carrying out surgery in tents was not appropriate in Gaza. Between October 2009 and April 2010, a series of meetings took place during which Hamas voiced a number of criticisms and demands. The criticisms focused on MSF's recruitment policy and the fact that it was not sufficiently integrated into public facilities, while the demands were related to access to patients' personal files and home visits by medical teams. As far as Hamas was concerned, MSF had to become an integral part of its planned re-organisation of public health facilities in order to "avoid duplication and wasting money".[4] It believed that incorporating the organisation into its public facilities would also allow the transfer of competencies to ministry staff. It also felt that, as no agreement had been signed with the ministry on surgical activities (intensive care unit and operating theatre), it could not guarantee the quality of care for which it deemed itself responsible. With regard to recruitment, MSF was accused of employing the ministry's surgeons without its knowledge and paying them much more than they received from the ministry as public sector employees. Two surgeons had indeed been hired by MSF in 2008. They were paid on a piecework basis and the increase in the number of interventions carried out after Operation Cast Lead meant they were earning up to 8,000 dollars a month. Lastly, the ministry demanded that MSF, like the other medical organisations working in Gaza, should stop making home visits and hand over the patients' full medical files so it could carry out the necessary follow-up in the event of complaints about medical treatment.

These criticisms of a legal and administrative nature were compounded by other factors. During the discussions between MSF and Hamas, frequent references were made to the behaviour of the teams, both national and international, and to "parties" held at MSF's offices where Palestinians mixed with expatriates and alcohol was consumed. This was "not how [Hamas] wished society to be organised".[5] Marked by Bernard Kouchner's statement and its rejection by the western world, Hamas also continued to express doubts about MSF's neutrality. It took issue with the weekly security meetings—intended to update the teams on travel conditions—which it saw as information-gathering sessions. In September 2009, two MSF employees were summoned by the internal security services and subjected to tough interrogation about MSF's work. However, their main criticism seemed to be directed at conduct outside of work, which they considered to be incompatible with the new social order that Hamas was endeavouring to establish.

These areas of dissension were a reflection of Hamas' determination to be recognised as the legitimate health authority in the Gaza Strip. Meanwhile, the Ministry of Health in Ramallah was still asking MSF to sign framework agreements and provide it with "information on its activities".[6]

At the end of 2009, the authors of MSF's strategic plan recognised the need to react to the new political and administrative reality in Gaza. "We will continue ongoing discussions with the authorities in the Gaza Strip to try to negotiate the freedom to get on with our work (Hamas is clearly determined to maintain strict control within the Strip). Our presence in Gaza will therefore depend on the compromises Hamas asks us to make".[7] But many of Hamas' demands were rapidly deemed legitimate as they emanated from a sovereign authority. The organisation undertook not to recruit any more health workers from the public sector and to provide Hamas with more information on the project. It also undertook to draw up a global agreement defining the framework of its intervention and to develop the plastic surgery project it wanted to set up in Nasser hospital in collaboration with the Gaza Ministry of Health. However, MSF refused to hand over the full patient files, citing its duty to respect medical confidentiality. The ministry finally agreed that this information should only be shared between doctors from MSF and the Ministry of Health. It also gave way on the issue of incorporating MSF's psychological and post-operative care facilities into the public system. MSF had argued that there was a danger of the confidentiality of information concerning patients receiving psychological care being jeopardised and that the choice of patients requiring physiotherapy should remain MSF's responsibility. However, the organisation promised that ministry staff would be offered physiotherapy training and agreed to stop home visits for functional rehabilitation and mental health patients at the end of February 2010.

These events highlight the difficulties encountered by MSF in adapting to the political changes in Gaza and to the demands being made by the new authorities with regard to health policy. Clinging to the belief that power over Gaza was still being exercised from Ramallah, the teams reacted relatively slowly in dealing with the new political authorities; this is viewed as one of the weaknesses in the action carried out by the organisation since 2006. There is no written evidence of an explicit choice being made by MSF, but based on a series of personal accounts by international staff, managers at headquarters and Palestinian employees,[8] there appear to be two reasons for this attitude. Firstly, the national team, recruited when Fatah was in power in Gaza and composed essentially of people close to Fatah and to left-wing Palestinian nationalist parties, probably influenced the way the international teams perceived events in the Gaza Strip. Secondly, it is likely that this influence was even more potent because most of the involved expatriates and project managers, including those at headquarters, had already accepted the prevailing representations of Palestinian political actors and accorded more legitimacy to the Palestinian movement that had signed the Oslo Accords, embodied by the Palestinian Authority and its main component, Fatah, than to Hamas. This ideological proximity, although doubtlessly implicit, combined with the perspective from which MSF was viewing the situation, goes some way to explaining why MSF found it so hard to alter its reading of what was happening in Gaza.

MSF saw the Hamas government as wishing to impose both health policy choices and its own vision of society and did not want to be dictated to on how it should behave and how it should run its activities. This stance was due partly to a political desire to limit its collaboration with Hamas and partly to its difficulty in understanding the deep mutations underway in Gaza. The organisation gave the ruling authorities the impression that it had put itself beyond their reach at a time when there was a real need to organise services for the population and consolidate their legitimacy.

Hamas finally left MSF no choice but to negotiate the scope of the organisation's operations in the Gaza Strip. These negotiations focused on both medical and administrative issues. However, after the political and military defeat of Fatah, its long-standing interlocutor in the Gaza Strip, MSF's relations with Israel were to be determined by matters of a completely different nature.

Israel and the Humanitarian Management of the Gaza Strip

Israel had evacuated its settlers and the military from the Gaza Strip in August 2005 as part of a non-negotiated withdrawal. However, it continued to control all entries and exits. For MSF, maintaining its activities therefore depended to a large extent on its relations with the Israeli authorities. This was all the more true after the Gaza blockade had been set up which, in theory, allowed through certain essential goods and humanitarian aid. In reality, however, orders of medical supplies and medicines sometimes remained stranded for days or even weeks if all the necessary permits hadn't been obtained, or if the contents of the crates contravened some aspect of the relatively vague rules governing the embargo—or even for no apparent reason.

The Israeli "Cast Lead" offensive was a perfect illustration of the role Israel intended humanitarian aid to play in Gaza. It also goes some way to explaining the relations between MSF and Israel, which was anxious to demonstrate its concern for humanitarian issues. Thus, in response to a French proposal for a "48-hour ceasefire on humanitarian grounds" on 1 January 2009, and in spite of the fact that 400 people on the Palestinian side had already been killed, the Israeli foreign minister, Tzipi Livni, explained that "aid convoys [were] being allowed through the border crossings" and that consequently there was "no humanitarian crisis in Gaza and [...] no need for a truce". When, on 31 May 2010, the Israeli army attacked a flotilla of six ships transporting humanitarian aid to Gaza, Israel's deputy ambassador to the United Nations, whose task it was to defend the blockade, took the same position, thereby minimising the consequences of the "strategy designed to throttle Gaza" that had been adopted by successive Israeli governments.[9]

Interviewed in early 2011 about intervention opportunities for MSF during Operation Cast Lead, the head of NGO relations at the Israeli Defence Ministry and Coordinator of Governmental Activities in the Territories (COGAT) retrospectively justified the authorisations given to MSF in the following terms: "During operation 'Cast Lead' we authorised entry to any humanitarian operator providing real humanitarian assistance. We allowed MSF entry because we knew it would be useful. MSF asked us if it could take in tent hospitals, medicines and humanitarian workers. And nothing is more humanitarian than medical assistance. If your movements are coordinated with the Israeli Liaison Office (DCL) and you are providing medical assistance, why would we refuse authorisation? Some NGOs wanted to go in just to see what was happening, not to help, and that's why they were refused access".[10]

For MSF, along with other humanitarian organisations, difficulties in getting aid into Gaza increased once the embargo was in place. For the organisation, 2007 started badly even before the "Battle of Gaza", with an incident that had serious consequences for its action. On 17 April, during a trip to Jerusalem to attend a meeting with the coordination team, a Palestinian employee from Gaza was arrested for taking part in a "conspiracy" against Israel. In addition to the dramatic personal consequences of the incident, this arrest and subsequent conviction had numerous repercussions for MSF. Rumours circulated in Gaza that MSF had betrayed its employee and handed him over to the Israelis. In Israel, the organisation was the victim of a short but virulent press campaign during which it was accused of promoting terrorism.[11] For the authorities in Tel-Aviv, this episode was a real opportunity: not only was MSF's credibility undermined, but the risk of attack could be used as justification for restricting movements between the West Bank, Jerusalem and the Gaza Strip. Yet the organisation managed to keep up its activities, to the extent that some organisations who experienced more difficulty than MSF in obtaining travel permits at the Erez terminal[12] border crossing believed it was getting special treatment. The Association of International Development Agencies (AIDA) published a communiqué in December 2008 in which it referred to differences in treatment between organisations: "Consequently, the use of a "security" justification to restrict entry by NGO staff to Erez for over twenty consecutive days beginning the first week of November is not consistent with prior security responses. Furthermore, the granting of permission for entry to MSF, UN, and ICRC staff is also not consistent with the justification of "security"".[13] However, although MSF had very little scope for negotiation with Israel, it appeared to content itself with this. For example, it didn't ask for more access to Jerusalem for staff in Gaza, and vice versa, in a conflict where access and the free movement of goods and people were major issues.

In such conditions, is it possible for medical aid organisations such as MSF to avoid becoming the healthcare assistants of the occupying power? The issue of NGOs assisting the occupation was explicitly raised by the president of MSF in 2002: "Until now, international humanitarian aid has only played a peripheral role in this conflict, but there is a danger of it being expected to assume that of assistant prison guard at the centre of a pitiless system of domination and segregation. After the capacity for resistance of the Palestinian population, it is now the independence of foreign relief workers that is being put to the test".[14]

Left-wing Israeli intellectuals also questioned the role of humanitarian aid at a time when four-fifths of Gaza's population were reliant upon it.[15] In their opinion, it was serving to "suspend the catastrophe" and freed Israel from the obligation of finding a way out of the conflict. For Adi Ophir and Arielle Azoulay, "the normal operation [of humanitarian and human rights organisations] is an extension of the ruling apparatus, one of its branches, the one responsible for the suspension of the catastrophe and the creation of chronic disaster".[16] Dov Weiss-glas, adviser to Prime Minister Ehud Olmert, in an attempt in early 2006 to justify the blockade after Hamas' victory in the legislative elections, commented: "It's like an appointment with the dietician. The Palestinians will get a lot thinner, but they won't die".[17] Some Palestinians also criticised the presence of NGOs in the occupied territories, believing that assistance programmes helped "normalise" the situation and relieved Israel of its responsibilities as the occupying power.

It should be noted that this notion that humanitarian aid can potentially collude with an oppressive system is not, however, confined to the Palestinian Territories. Furthermore, MSF has only a minor role in the aid operations conducted in the Territories in general, and in Gaza in particular.

There are settings in which it is hard to avoid polarisation, and the Palestinian Territories is one of them. MSF has only ever worked with the Palestinian population and never in Israel, something that it is reproached for on occasion in the Israeli press. Consequently, the issue of its "neutrality" in the Israeli-Palestinian conflict has often been raised. It has also been raised with regard to its relations with the two Palestinian political factions, especially as, after the violent transfer of power between Fatah and Hamas in Gaza, its teams were confronted with what was for them a whole new scenario.

The imbalance in the forces involved, the media attention attracted by the conflict which offered countless opportunities for public statements, the proximity of the international teams to the Palestinian staff, as well as their daily exposure to the conflict, made political neutrality difficult and fostered the international teams' empathy with the Palestinians, whom they perceived as victims. In 2001, the subject was discussed in a board meeting: "Many of them [members of the field team] are asking why their testimony gathering is not being reported by MSF; why we are not publically denouncing Israel's policies and practices in the Palestinian Territories". It was in response to these demands that MSF began publishing its "Palestinian chronicles"[18] in 2002. Presented as "an account of the day-to-day reality of a population trapped by war and whose suffering is largely ignored", these chronicles contained the highlights of MSF's testimony activity in the Territories and helped soothe tensions between the field teams and headquarters.

Recordings of discussions at board level reveal that several members of the team were considered to be "overly-invested in 'testimony' gathering".[19] Bearing witness to the living conditions of the Palestinians and to the violence they were suffering had become an end in itself for some of the team who expected to see MSF make its position public. Yet the organisation acknowledged that the requirement for "neutrality" was pushed to the limit when, as remarked by its president: "The military occupation is accompanied by such violence against the inhabitants of the Territories, the balance of power is so unequal, that there is a certain indulgence of the weakest, even when they commit crimes".[20]

A few years later, the programme managers raised the issue again in very similar terms: "Are we neutral? We don't expect individuals to be completely neutral given their proximity to the Palestinians and the frequent imbalances in the conflict, but the organisation itself must use neutral language. We expect international staff (and, as far as possible, national staff) to try to maintain a certain degree of objectivity, to avoid biased and critical language and to stick to the facts".[21] The support by some of the teams for the secular and national programme of Yasser Arafat's party, the recruitment of employees ideologically close to Fatah or to left-wing parties, an intervention initially designed for a situation opposing Palestinians and Israelis—and not two Palestinian factions—were all factors that contributed to make the political transition in Gaza a perilous experience for MSF.

Translated from French by Mandy Duret

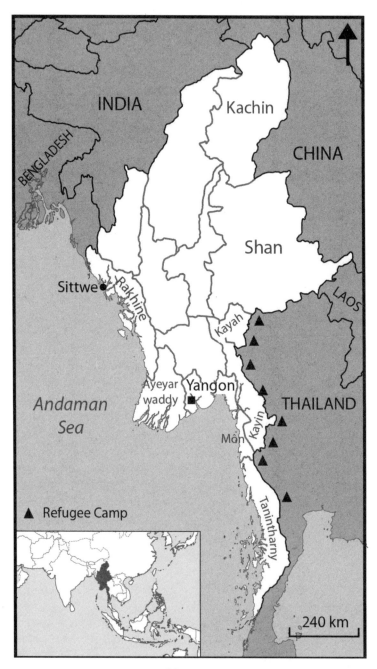

Myanmar

MYANMAR

"GOLFING WITH THE GENERALS"

Fiona Terry[1]

Whether or not international aid organisations should operate in the repressive, authoritarian state of Myanmar provokes passionate debate. On one side are many exile groups and their supporters—predominantly based in Thailand, the US and the UK—who argue that it is impossible to provide aid inside Myanmar without strengthening the military regime. On the other side are aid organisations that have chosen to work inside the country. They argue that aid can be delivered responsibly and reach people in need of assistance without undue advantage to the junta. The debate is acrimonious and brings out half-truths on both sides: the exile groups exaggerate the regime's excesses and the benefits accrued from international aid, and in-country agencies, in response, downplay the constraints imposed on them by the military regime.

The experience of Médecins Sans Frontières in Myanmar falls squarely within this polemic. The French section of MSF withdrew from the country in 2006 after five years of efforts to mount an effective malaria treatment programme in conflict-affected areas bordering

Thailand. It publicly denounced "the unacceptable conditions imposed by the authorities" which, if accepted, would render MSF "nothing more than a technical service provider subject to the political priorities of the junta".[2] At the other end of the spectrum lies the Dutch section of MSF which runs the largest medical programme of any aid organisation in Myanmar. It treats twice as many AIDS patients as the government and all aid agencies combined, and runs clinics across four of the country's states and divisions.[3] Somewhere in between these positions, wracked with uncertainty, sits the Swiss section of MSF. It has faced major impediments to its projects since it intervened in 1999, but chose to quietly challenge government restrictions and persevere with its medical programmes.

The common explanation—whispered in the corridors of aid offices in Yangon and throughout the MSF movement—for the Dutch section's success operating in this authoritarian state is that "the head of MSF-H plays golf with the generals". Like all good rumours, it is part based on fact. Unable to secure a meeting with the regional commander to discuss opening a clinic in a mining area of Kachin State, the head of MSF-Holland visited the golf club in Myitkyina where he knew the commander to be playing, and asked for his authorisation. The request was granted and MSF established the clinic. In the moralistic tones often employed in the aid world, particularly in MSF, this story grew into a generalised myth that the head of MSF-Holland—who stayed an unprecedented fifteen years in the same post—had special relations with certain generals and was for all intents and purposes "a collaborator". The person in question did little to dispel the myth, avoiding debate on activities proposed, rejecting suggestions of public advocacy construed as critical of the regime, and publicly denying the difficulties of operating in Myanmar.

Nevertheless, that "playing golf" has become a euphemism for "collaboration" is indicative of a broader difficulty all MSF sections faced adapting their principles and methods of working to the Myanmar context. After all, playing golf is a small price to pay for good relations with a commander who determines what MSF can and cannot do for the population. It might be different were MSF asked to buy the commander golf clubs, or renew his club membership. But rather than analysing how MSF-Holland mounted this ambitious programme in such a difficult context and questioning the methods employed, all MSF sections, including the Dutch section's headquarters in Amsterdam, preferred to stick with, and then turn a blind eye to, the fallacy of an unhealthy and privileged relationship.

This chapter explores the political choices made by the three MSF sections in response to the constraints and dilemmas they faced working in Myanmar. How could two sections of the same organisation have reached such different conclusions over the ability to work in a country? What were the compromises made and strategies pursued by each that lead to such different levels of engagement with the Myanmar people?

The Choice to Intervene

Having no official mandate to determine the types of situations to which it ought to respond, MSF freely chooses where it will and will not offer its humanitarian medical assistance. The French section of MSF began working with refugees from the Karen ethnic group in Thailand in early 1984 and was active until the 2000s in villages and camps along the border and in running cross-border operations into territory held by the rebel Karen National Union (KNU). Although the refugee context was highly politicised, it seemed less problematic to assist victims of the junta outside the country than from within. So when MSF-Holland requested authorisation to enter Myanmar in 1989, it faced considerable scepticism from within the MSF movement.

The Dutch section's primary rationale for intervening was to investigate health needs in border areas beset by armed conflict, and to be a witness for the outside world of what was going on.[4] The Myanmar army was conducting brutal counterinsurgency campaigns in several ethnic states bordering Thailand, Laos and China, which aimed to deprive insurgents of a support base by forcing villagers to move to government-controlled settlements and razing their homes and crops. Reports of rape, forced conscription and labour, and summary executions circulated among the communities of 140,000 refugees who escaped to Thailand. Less was known about the hardships faced in Kachin State bordering China, where the Dutch section initially wished to go. Speaking publicly about the causes of suffering constituted an important element in MSF's desire to intervene.

Repression elsewhere in Myanmar also "qualified" the country for MSF's attention. Northern Rakhine State is home to Muslim Rohingyas and smaller Hindu minorities who are denied citizenship, and as such are more vulnerable than most to the arbitrary abuse of power by Myanmar officials. Harsh laws govern almost every aspect of their lives, from the age at which they may marry to whether they may travel outside their home village, with sometimes dire consequences for their ability to access medical services. Unlike the Karen and Mon in Thailand, most Rohingyas who fled state repression were not given sanctuary in a neighbouring country, but were twice pushed back from Bangladesh, once in 1978, and again in 1994–95. They returned to similar repression and brutality from which they had fled, exacerbated for many by the seizure of land and property by the government in their absence. Both the Dutch and French sections of MSF worked with the refugees in Bangladesh and were vocal critics of the government's refoulement to Myanmar and the complicity of the UNHCR in the process.[5]

In addition to the border conflicts and generalised repression, the Myanmar people suffer from a state of abject poverty brought about by the incompetence and investment priorities of the junta, which are sharply skewed towards maintaining power and military might over internal and external enemies—both real and imagined. This is especially felt in the health sector, on which a staggeringly low 0.3% of GDP is spent. Millions of people do not have access to affordable and effective healthcare, and are vulnerable to suffer and die from preventable and treatable diseases such as malaria. Myanmar faces one of the worst HIV epidemics in Asia and among the worst TB prevalence rates in the world. Inadequate treatment is causing multidrug-resistance to TB, with repercussions that are likely to be felt well beyond Myanmar's borders.

Thus there was no shortage of serious health problems to justify MSF's attempts to work in Myanmar. Although the country has rarely experienced an acute emergency in which large numbers of people were at risk of imminent death (the obvious exception being in the aftermath of Cyclone Nargis in 2008), the "chronic emergency" from which its population suffers is extremely widespread. The problem with intervening lay less in the "what to do" than the "how to do it". How can MSF assure that in helping the victims, it does not inadvertently strengthen the hand of their oppressors?

Entering the Country

Right from the outset, MSF-Holland faced a major hurdle in its efforts to, quite literally, get a footing in Myanmar. Its request to work there in 1989 was prompted by a small opening in the regime's isolationist stance which, until then, had limited the presence of aid organisations to a handful of UN agencies and the ICRC. In the wake of international condemnation of the crackdown on pro-democracy demonstrators in 1988 and the imposition of sanctions by many western governments, the regime took a few steps to improve its image, including opening the door a crack to international NGOs. But in an early prelude to demands made after Cyclone Nargis, the military regime was prepared to accept foreign aid but no MSF personnel on its soil. This was a condition that MSF could not accept—it would be impossible to assess needs or monitor the use of aid without the presence of foreign staff. It took two years of negotiations before an international staff member was authorised to stay in the then capital, Yangon. He arrived in January 1992.

In an effort to distance itself from the activities of MSF in Thailand and Bangladesh, MSF-Holland adopted the Dutch version of its name, Artzen Zonder Grenzen (AZG) for use inside the country—a name by which it is still known today (and hereafter will be used). It also entered Myanmar under the auspices of UNICEF, setting up an office in the same building and using UNICEF's "good name" to establish its credentials.[6] Although the use of "AZG" continues to raise eyebrows in the MSF movement, this was a small price to pay for access if it was indeed the difference in name that shielded AZG from the scrutiny to which MSF-France was subjected when it sought permission to work in-country in 1995. The health minister supported the French section's request but the higher echelons of the military rejected it, allegedly due to MSF's cross-border activities and association with the KNU.

It took a much larger opening in the regime's attitude to the exterior before MSF-France was able to return to Myanmar in 2000. By this stage MSF-Switzerland had also opted to enter Myanmar, having undertaken an exploratory assessment in 1998 at the invitation of the Health Ministry. At this time, international aid organisations were surfing on a wave of unprecedented—albeit relative—openness, instigated by the number three of the regime, Khin Nyunt. The junta had opened its prisons, labour camps and some border areas to the ICRC's scrutiny, and AZG and other NGOs were expanding operations. The honeymoon was not to last.

Negotiating Humanitarian Activities

Once inside the country, all MSF sections faced constraints as to what they were allowed to do, necessitating some difficult choices and trade-offs between competing objectives. There were three main areas of compromise that each section made on their ideal ways of working: in their independence to choose where and with whom to work; in their ability to fully control and monitor their aid; and in their ability to speak freely about the underlying causes of health problems in the country.

Independence of Choice

The mistrustful atmosphere into which AZG landed in 1992 did not bode well for much freedom of movement or choice of target population. During the long period of negotiations to enter the country, AZG's attention focused on the plight of Rohingyas in Rakhine State, following a government crackdown on dissent in 1991 and 1992 which provoked 250,000 to flee to Bangladesh. But access to Rakhine State was not what the government had in mind, and in its first year AZG was directed towards providing healthcare in Shwepyithar township on the outskirts of Yangon. AZG agreed to this proposal for "strategic" reasons, as a "foot-in-the-door" through which to build relationships of trust with officials, and encourage openings in areas with more pressing needs.

AZG was soon confronted with knowledge of a more impoverished township built on paddy fields across the river from Yangon called Hlaing Thayar. In an early test of whether it could, at least at the local level, prioritise assistance to those most in need, AZG requested permission to include Hlaing Thayar in a nutritional survey planned for Shwepyithar in July 1992. In what was a promising sign of AZG's negotiating potential, the government accepted, and high rates of malnutrition found among children helped to convince the authorities to allow AZG to assist both townships.

Yet, these townships were no ordinary suburbs of Yangon but were areas to which residents of dozens of shanty-towns were forcibly relocated after the regime burned down their homes in the wake of the 1988 student uprising. The shanty-towns had provided a ready source of protesters to join street demonstrations, and passageways through which they could escape capture by police, and so the government wanted them destroyed and cared little for the welfare of their occupants. Fifty thousand "squatters" were moved to Hlaing Thayar in 1989, a figure which had swelled to 164,000 by 1995.[7] AZG did not fully recognise the dilemma it faced, one which is recurrent in situations of forced relocation. By providing healthcare to the displaced, AZG certainly eased their hardship. But by its presence and participation in the government-run system, AZG was tacitly condoning the government's forced relocation policy, especially as relocations continued despite AZG's presence.

The Dutch section did express concern at the forced relocations, raising the health implications with government interlocutors, and showing visiting donors the townships to help expose the regime's practices.[8] But as I discuss later, the impact of lobbying for change within the regime and particularly through outsiders was extremely limited. Had AZG eluded government controls and forged decent relations with the population, perhaps a stronger case for its presence could be made. In an indictment of the limits imposed, one programme review from 1996 recommended holding talks with the highest levels of the Health Department to establish whether an MSF staff member, facing an emergency at the hospital when there was no other doctor or nurse present, was permitted to save a life. "Or should s/he just note down what s/he observes and let the patient die?"[9]

AZG did not lose sight of its target population, and its persistence paid off when it was allowed to visit Rakhine State in April 1993. It was not permitted independent access, but was accompanied by Ministry of Health officials in addition to a police escort for outlying areas. AZG wanted to work in the predominantly Muslim townships from which the highest proportion of refugees in Bangladesh had fled and to which many were returning, but it again had to compromise on its choice of location, obliged to base itself in the state capital, Sittwe. Given that malaria was the leading pathology in Rakhine State, AZG set up a malaria control programme which included training microscopists to diagnose malaria, prevention activities and treatment. AZG also ran mobile malaria clinics in nine townships, which exposed the teams to some of the problems of discrimination and forced labour meted out to the inhabitants of the region. But according to one project coordinator, AZG's primary goal of advocacy on behalf of the Rohingyas soon gave way to a medical focus. "Although this time was spent travelling in Rakhine, the emphasis was very much on high quality medical and laboratory activities and very little seems to have been reported or written down about the political or advocacy aspects of Rakhine".[10] It took another four years before AZG was finally permitted to establish a base in the Muslim enclave of Maungdaw, in January 1998.

An attempt to expand operations to conflict-affected populations in Kachin State ended in last-minute failure in 1995 when AZG did not present the local commander with a personal gift as another NGO had done. But impediments on the political front during this time began to be offset by unexpected successes on the medical front, reorientating AZG's approach from the "foot-in-the-door" confidence-building efforts to one of "medical diplomacy"—acquiring leverage through its medical expertise and operational volume. The break-through came when AZG was pseudo-officially permitted to carry out a malaria drug-resistance study in Rakhine State with Health Ministry staff in late 1995, which showed the ineffectiveness of the national treatment protocol.[11] The health minister was furious when he saw the publication, but by that time AZG had received permission from lower down to change treatment in Rakhine State from chloroquine and sulphadoxine-pyrimethamine to mefloquine artesunate. When a civilian medical doctor took over as deputy health minister in 2001, the protocol officially changed to the more effective treatment. Through "medical diplomacy" the Dutch section was also instrumental in breaking the taboo over mention of the growing AIDS epidemic in Myanmar, and received permission to start health education and condom distributions in Hlaing Thayar township. Pushing for more, AZG started to care openly for people living with AIDS, both treating opportunistic infections and addressing the widespread stigmatisation of AIDS sufferers through social programmes. Then in August 2003, AZG pioneered treatment of AIDS patients in Myanmar with antiretroviral drugs, challenging the prevailing dogma among health agencies that in-country capacity was too low to allow for little more than health education and social marketing of condoms.[12] Within five years, AZG was providing over 10,000 patients with these life-saving drugs.

This pragmatic shift to a medical focus reorientated AZG's target population from those affected by repression or armed conflict to those affected by deadly disease. Malaria clinics, once "alibi projects" to gain access to certain areas, were joined by sexually transmitted disease

(STD), HIV and tuberculosis treatment programmes to become ends in themselves. From the late 1990s, project areas were selected by the vulnerability of inhabitants to infectious diseases: (STD) clinics were opened in the jade-mining areas of Kachin State to reduce transmission of venereal disease, and hence HIV, among the itinerant population, sex workers and intravenous drug users. AZG began harm reduction and needle exchange activities, and increased health education about the causes and consequences of HIV infection. Similar projects began in Shan State. With a virus rather than army brutality as the cause, together with growing concern at its spread, the regime placed fewer impediments in the way of AZG's requests to establish clinics in new areas. This shift proved to be a shrewd political choice that dramatically increased the number of people AZG was able to assist.

Turning to the Swiss section of MSF (MSF-CH), it also had to compromise on its choice of location when it first entered the country in 1999. Although it gave a medical reason—among the highest rates of drug-resistant malaria in the world—as its rationale for wanting to work in the three states of Kayin, Mon and Kayah that border Thailand, MSF-CH had to start work in the coastal region of Tanintharyi Division. "We had to compromise from the beginning and accept to sacrifice our independence with regards to where we wanted to work", remembers the first head of mission, Patrick Wieland. "We thought that little-by-little we would gain the confidence of the local authorities and gradually reach the border regions". But the strategy was only partially successful.

We did gain some ground towards the border with malaria mobile clinics, but we were never able to put a fixed clinic where we wanted to. We pushed to get as close as we could and people would come, sometimes from up to 40 kilometres away, to access our clinics.[13]

As the country continued to open under the influence of Khin Nyunt, MSF-CH obtained access to Kayah State, something no other aid organisation, including the ICRC, had managed beyond visiting the state prison. The Swiss section established a fixed clinic north of the state capital, Loikaw, in March 2004. In the everyday frustrations and constraints of working in Myanmar, simply establishing a base was considered a major achievement in "opening humanitarian space", even though MSF-CH was unable to reach conflict-affected areas of Kayah State where it assumed—on the basis of reports by border-based agencies—that thousands of civilians were in need of humanitarian assistance. It had to be content that it was at least providing a primary healthcare clinic to which people displaced by the army could come and receive treatment. From that base, MSF-CH kept pressing for authorisation to move closer to areas of low-level conflict with mobile clinics and through its partnership with a local NGO, Karuna.

The French section, when it started programmes in 2001, did not face the same dilemma as MSF-CH and MSF-H in having to begin operations in a different area to that which it proposed. It began a project to improve diagnosis and treatment of malaria, first in Mon and later in Kayin State, through both fixed and mobile clinics, also pushing the limits of areas to which it was authorised to go, often by boat. MSF made large improvements in the medical care of malaria patients in the first year: the case fatality rate among hospitalised malaria patients in Mudon halved between July 2001 and June 2002, and no malaria deaths occurred in the hospital in the second half of 2002.[14] Furthermore, the "foot-in-the-door" approach worked to a certain extent, with projects permitted to expand into new areas such as Ye Township and Kayin State. In the newly accessible areas, the 7,500 consultations held between April and August 2004 exceeded predictions for the entire year.[15] This convinced MSF of the need to continue to expand activities towards the border, eventually perhaps to link up with cross-border activities from Thailand. But the purge of Prime Minister Khin Nyunt and his entire military intelligence apparatus in October 2004 sounded the death knell for further expansion for several years.

Control and Monitoring of Aid

The second main compromise the MSF sections made in Myanmar was to relinquish control over their ability to monitor the use of aid at all times. The government periodically imposed tight restrictions on travel to project sites—sometimes affecting only foreign personnel, sometimes all staff—which hindered the supervision of MSF's projects. As shown above, travel restrictions had long been a feature of working in Myanmar, but these intensified after the purge of Khin Nyunt in an effort to reign in the aid agencies that had expanded operations on his authority. Hardliners replaced more moderate ministers in the government and controls over aid organisations increased: limits on the length of time allowed outside Yangon; prior approval of all new expatriate staff; lists of national staff submitted regularly to the government; lengthy process of registration with a central and line ministry; and more frequent renegotiations of the Memorandums of Understanding (MoU). Aid agencies were also obliged to take a government "liaison officer" with them on every field trip, which had to be organised weeks in advance.

All sections of MSF had to weigh up the effects of these rules on their ability to control and monitor the use of aid, versus what they were still able to do and might be able to do if they persevered. Contrary to claims of some exile groups, government diversion of aid—the common fear when unable to properly monitor its use—was never of serious concern. Unlike the government-sponsored scams seen in North Korea or Ethiopia, any theft of aid that did take place was done at the local, individual level: an area commander commandeering a boat or car for his personal use; the local Township Medical Officer stealing drugs for his private clinic; or Ministry of Health staff selling polio vaccines rather than providing them free of charge.[16] Although frustrating in themselves, the scale of these problems was a far cry from government-sanctioned taxation or the re-direction of aid to "worthy" groups seen elsewhere. It is the fungibility of aid that caused more discomfort than its diversion per se: all MSF programmes assume responsibilities in the health field that should be the remit of government, thereby allowing state resources to be directed elsewhere. Many MSF staff expressed their unease at this, although less so at the macro level, since few believe that the government would allocate more to the health sector if MSF left—the callous disregard shown by the regime towards Nargis survivors in proceeding with the referendum while they buried their dead, put pay to any lingering doubts about the government's priorities. Rather, this dilemma was felt more acutely at the local level where MSF's efforts to avoid collaborating with the regime resulted in the establishment of independent health structures—sometimes only metres from a government clinic—further undermining local capacity.[17]

The increased controls over aid activities that followed the purge of Khin Nyunt in late 2004 affected each MSF section differently. MSF-CH projects in Kayah State and Tanintharyi Division were deemed off-limits for months on end. MSF-CH persevered with the endless bureaucratic procedures now needed to get staff in-country, only to have them blocked in Yangon. Some even finished their assignment without ever having reached their project site.[18] The waste of money and human resources this entailed reignited long-standing debates in MSF-CH over whether it should remain in Myanmar or leave. In the end, it was the "stay" view that prevailed, carried by the argument that MSF could not abandon the 500 patients it had recently put on antiretroviral drugs. To do so would be to sentence them to death. Hence in many ways, MSF-CH became hostage to their AIDS treatment programme, changing the parameters of what the section would and would not accept to compromise on in Myanmar.

MSF-France, which did not have any patients on ARV treatment, decided to the contrary. The latest wave of restrictions came just as MSF had finally negotiated a permanent base in Ye from which to expand medical coverage. The regime put a stop to it all, preventing any potential witnesses to its crackdown on insurgents and those deemed to support them. The French section withdrew in March 2006, with the programme manager explaining:

"For humanitarian organisations, the issue is to recognize when our role has been reduced to being a technical service provider of the Myanmar authorities, subject to their political agenda and no longer to the goals that we have set for ourselves as a humanitarian organisation. Speaking for the French section's programmes, we believe that we have crossed that line. It is with great bitterness that we have had to decide to leave the country".[19]

But even in leaving, MSF-France made a final compromise, stifling its tendencies to rally public opinion and stoke debate about the limits of humanitarian action in such a context.

The Sound of Silence

The French section's relatively low-key departure subscribed within the logic of self-censorship that marked the third main compromise MSF sections made in Myanmar. "Witnessing" and "speaking out" (*témoignage* in French) had become an important part of MSF's action since the 1980s.[20] By mobilising public opinion and political players, MSF aims to pressure for change. But in Myanmar, all sections believed that any public comments construed as critical of the regime would jeopardise operations, to the detriment of hundreds of thousands of patients that MSF treats annually. The teams also worried about the safety of national staff if MSF were to incur the wrath of the regime.

For these—and several other reasons related to internal organisational changes at MSF in Paris—the French section left in a half-hearted manner. AZG and MSF-CH have seldom commented publicly on the causes of suffering and constraints to addressing it—except in relation to insufficient AIDS treatment and only then in 2008[21]—in all their years of operation.

Treating the symptoms of repression while unable to address the causes produced discomfort among AZG staff. AZG had intervened in Myanmar to be a witness for the outside world, yet without much discussion or debate, had mounted a medical programme that could be jeopardised by any criticism of the regime's policies and practices. The obvious tension between the more advocacy-oriented "humanitarian affairs" department (HAD) in Amsterdam and the coordination team in Yangon gave rise to incoherence in programmes and objectives. The HAD produced in-depth internal papers on the plight of the Rohingya and instructed field teams to collect and compile data on incidents, which were shared behind closed doors with donors and non-operational agencies working on these issues. But without a consistent purpose for the data collection over the long years, efforts waxed and waned. It is difficult to discern whether, in fact, the purpose was more about improving the situation for the Rohingya or fulfilling a self-prescribed "duty" of MSF to "witness and speak out". The disconnect between the perspectives of Yangon and Amsterdam is well illustrated in the Myanmar policy papers from 2001 to 2009, produced at headquarters. Yangon's bottom line was clearly determined by its medical programme: it was not going to jeopardise its ability to treat 200,000 malaria patients in Rakhine State each year. Yet Amsterdam clung to the belief that witnessing was the primary reason for which AZG should stay in Myanmar.

There might be more that AZG could do to try to ease hardships for the Rohingya if the medical and "advocacy" components of the programme were more in sync. Documenting, compiling and reporting in private to the relevant authorities on impediments to healthcare—such as travel restrictions impeding referrals and the prohibitive cost of passing through checkpoints—could be a less threatening way to bring about change than public statements on these issues, and more effective than back-door discussions with donors.

Influencing the Myanmar regime's behaviour is notoriously difficult. Richard Horsey, former head of the International Labour Organisation's office in Myanmar, describes the regime's strange contradiction that works against both back-door and public pressure:

[The regime] is at once dismissive of outside criticism, but at the same time curiously sensitive about how it is perceived. It seems to genuinely believe it is acting in the national interest, and feels deeply misunderstood, and unfairly treated, by the world at large.[22]

On the one hand, this dismissiveness limits the leverage and influence of external powers, even fellow Asian states, on the regime's behaviour, rendering futile the efforts of aid organisations to get Myanmar's allies to pressure for improvements. On the other hand, the regime's sensitivity to its image provokes a backlash when it is publicly criticised. The generals expelled the head of the UN, Charles Petrie, in October 2007 after he dared suggest in his UN Day speech that the government was not doing enough to address basic human needs. Petrie also raised the monk-led "saffron revolt" of a month earlier, saying "the concerns of the people have been clearly expressed through the recent peaceful demonstrations—it is beholden on all to listen".[23] This statement came in the wake of several other public criticisms from agencies working in the country, beginning with the ICRC's rare public denunciation of a government in June 2007,which accused Myanmar of major and repeated violations of international humanitarian law. The ICRC condemned the use of detainees as porters for the army, and lamented the regime's refusal to engage in dialogue or to allow the institution independent access to prisons.[24] A few months later, thirteen NGOs issued a joint statement calling on the government to ease restrictions on their attempts to help the poorest.[25] Petrie's expulsion quelled further outbursts, and the ICRC's continued absence from prisons or border areas provides a reminder of the resistance of the regime to all outside influence and pressure.

Neither MSF section lent their support to these initiatives which publicly questioned the regime's practices. They adopted a more discreet approach, challenging the rules through actions rather than words. Both sections frequently work without proper authorisation, sending teams of national staff to assess the needs of the newly displaced and working for long periods without a valid MoU. They also engage with outlawed groups like sex-workers and drug users, which carries risk of imprisonment for MSF's national staff, and work on the basis that it is better to apologise after the fact than be denied permission from the outset. In the wake of Cyclone Nargis, for example,

AZG did not await permission to send a team to the delta region. Its Bangladeshi and Chinese doctors managed to remain inconspicuous and stayed on long after all other foreigners were told to leave. MSF-CH has developed a strategy of "access by annoyance", repeatedly requesting authorisations to travel, constantly asking for explanations when denied permission, and reiterating time and again its desire to reach those most in need. MSF-CH also sent teams and medical supplies to the sites of street protests during the saffron revolt in 2007 and tried to help the injured, even becoming blocked inside Sule Pagoda at the centre of Yangon when the area was cordoned off by police.[26] Although largely symbolic in its impact—injured protesters were probably afraid of visibility if treated by foreigners so stayed away—MSF-CH felt this show of solidarity was important, especially in the absence of assistance from other organisations except the ICRC.[27]

But for all these acts of "resistance" and the number of patients treated, it is hard not to wonder whether MSF has become too mechanical in its approach, too detached from the context—seeing people in terms of the illnesses they bear rather than who they are and what they are suffering in the larger sense. A recent programme evaluation speaks of the Rakhine project as sclerotic:[28] that despite early successes in changing protocols and influencing acceptance of HIV in the country, AZG has not used its sizeable weight enough to push for change, which could include easing travel restrictions on patient referrals.

Whilst it is understandable that MSF prioritises operational presence over public criticism in Myanmar when so little might be gained and so much lost by the latter, it is less so to hear what is said publicly—downplaying the constraints faced by aid organisations, and showing little solidarity with those who would rather change the system and do away with the need for international aid, than merely accept its handouts. The polarised environment is partly to blame for the former, as any admission of difficulties is seized upon by activists and used in arguments against giving aid. But this does not justify the tone and extent of the denial. When asked in an interview what conditions MSF-CH has to accept in order to work in Myanmar, the head of mission mentioned only the MoU, and said that this was no different to what exists in other countries: "The military junta has the right to monitor our activities, exactly as the government would do in France". He blamed false rumours for concerns about working conditions for NGOs and claimed that MSF knows how to work in Myanmar: "We are very conscious of the practices going on in this country. We know what tone to adopt when we want to intervene in disaster areas, but we also know [how to] denounce when things don't work as they should". He ended the interview comparing the lives of the people to that of "almost all developing countries" and blamed the foreign media for "exaggerating" the poor living conditions of the Burmese.[29]

In a similar vein, the head of AZG showed a distinct lack of interest in the fate of injured monks and other protesters during the saffron revolt of October 2007. When asked by CNN whether AZG had a moral obligation to demand access to the injured and detained, the programme manager merely said, "If they come to us or if we know where they are we will treat them like anybody else". Evidently surprised by this response, the interviewer asked the question again. This time the response was more elaborate:

You see, we have a very large programme. We have treated last year more than one million patients, for malaria, AIDS. These programme activities are still going on. We are working for deadly diseases. So it is very important for us to continue the treatment of these patients and this is actually where our staff is busy in these clinics serving these more than a million people.[30]

AZG's shift from concern for victims to concern for "diseases" was complete.

What emerges from the analysis above is that the three sections of MSF pursued very different approaches towards working inside Myanmar, with varying success. AZG initially aimed to assist conflict-affected populations by speaking publicly about their plight, but after several years of failed attempts, greater success on the medical front, and a realisation that public advocacy is likely to prompt an end to its projects, switched its focus to the less controversial area of disease. Given the state of public health in Myanmar and the certain death awaiting those infected with HIV, severe malaria and multidrug-resistant TB, few could argue that this was not a legitimate choice. Moreover, by establishing clinics in high-risk mining areas, AZG probably assisted many displaced by conflict who migrated to these zones.

But the downside to AZG's approach is that it came at the cost of turning a blind eye to the larger picture. In the narrow focus and routine of the medical programmes, the context became "normal" and the unacceptable accepted, such as forced labour on the street outside a clinic or the crackdown on monks protesting in the street.

MSF-CH, for its part, pursued a relentless quest to access victims of the regime's brutal policies, which it assumed were found in the conflict-affected border regions. Incredible energy and resources were spent over four years trying to reach sensitive areas of Kayah State. Yet only one year after finally succeeding, MSF-CH transferred its programmes to another NGO for lack of patients. MSF-CH had been understandably reluctant to believe the junta's claims that few people remained in these areas, preferring to trust the population estimates given by border-based activist groups. But these turned out to be inflated, giving greater validity to AZG's choice to focus on areas to which the displaced might have gone, such as mining towns. As a consequence, MSF-CH is now following in the footsteps of AZG, tackling infectious diseases in its clinics and in Myanmar's prisons.

The French section's strategy, or lack thereof, in Myanmar was the most disappointing. The decision to close operations in Myanmar inspired little debate in Paris and, unlike in contexts such as the Rwandan refugee camps, no thought was given to how MSF's withdrawal might be used to the advantage of those aid agencies who chose to stay. Few were even informed. MSF-France lacked the imagination and passion it has shown elsewhere to find alternative ways of reaching the population, in defiance of the authorities. Instead of beefing up existing cross-border operations, the French ceased medical runs into Mon State and all but a small TB programme in the Thai camps. This was a far cry from MSF's determination to continue assisting North Koreans once it had withdrawn from the country in 1998, finding innovative ways to help refugees in China in spite of Beijing's opposition. Furthermore, in masking its operational inertia with claims to "have been gullible to have believed humanitarian space could exist in Myanmar",[31] MSF-France gave fuel to those arguing that international aid to the country should stop.

Critics of aid in Myanmar are incorrect when they suggest that aid is propping up the Myanmar regime, or that it is a uniquely difficult context in which to work. Nevertheless, aid organisations make some serious compromises when working in the country, particularly in relation to whom they are permitted to assist. Whilst MSF teams on the ground grapple with the dilemmas and difficulties they face, there seems to be little consistent discussion of parameters or benchmarks against which to judge acceptable from unacceptable compromises within any section and particularly across sections. MSF just drifts from one compromise or victory to the next without much assessment as to what worked and what did not, or any overall plan. Both MSF-CH and AZG are carrying out some remarkable work in the medical field, assisting large numbers of people. But rather than seeing this as an end in itself, MSF and especially AZG need to rethink how they can use this influence to improve the plight of people whose essential problem is not illness per se but the repression and deprivation at its source. The delicate challenge is to find a way to push for change without exposing patients, MSF staff and allies within the regime to punishment if falling foul of those in charge.

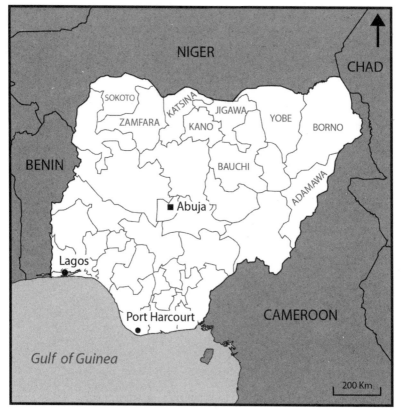

Nigeria

NIGERIA

PUBLIC (HEALTH) RELATIONS

Claire Magone[1]

It was via a dispatch published in early February 1996 by *Agence France-Presse* that MSF's French section in Paris (MSF-F) learnt of the meningitis epidemic affecting the north east and north west of Nigeria.[2] Deploying a new system of intervention "whose stated objective [was] to build a nationality-less team bearing the MSF label"[3] (the Emergency Team), MSF's operational sections in Amsterdam, Barcelona, Brussels and Paris organised a response to the epidemic on a scale unprecedented in the organisation's history: ninety international staff were sent out to the three worst-hit Nigerian states of Kano, Bauchi and Katsina where, between March and May 1996, they vaccinated 2.9 million people and treated 30,000 patients.

The operation allowed MSF to assert its legitimacy as a responder to epidemics in "open settings" ("closed settings" being displaced persons or refugee camps). This legitimacy was consolidated later in 1996 with an international symposium entitled "Operational Reponses to Epidemics in Developing Countries", organised to mark its 25th anniversary[4] and then, in collaboration with the WHO, UNICEF and the

International Federation of the Red Cross, the establishment in 1997 of the International Coordination Group (ICG). The purpose of the ICG was to ensure the availability of emergency supplies of meningococcal polysaccharide vaccines as world stocks had been exhausted by the epidemics in Nigeria. MSF's concern with epidemics echoed that of the WHO which devoted its 1996 world health report to the resurgence and emergence of new forms of infectious diseases, which it saw as announcing an imminent "global crisis".[5]

MSF's objective was to provide a response to the "epidemic of epidemics"[6] that its teams had been confronted with since the beginning of the 1990s: cholera in Mali, Côte d'Ivoire, Liberia, Cape Verde, Senegal and Somalia; yellow fever in Liberia, Ebola hemorrhagic fever in Zaire and meningitis in Niger. But this response would also provide the organisation with an opportunity. In the words of Philippe Biberson, president of MSF-France at the time, "aid to refugees currently concerns [...] only a tiny proportion of MSF's projects [...]; much of the know-how and experience we have gained is of little use to the missions we're developing now". Thus, responding to epidemics in open settings was a chance for MSF to develop new projects while continuing to deploy the medical and logistical expertise it had acquired in refugee camps.

But transferring its know-how from one intervention setting to another meant rethinking its relations with the national politico-administrative authorities. In exceptional settings, such as refugee camps, governments often keep their distance, delegating the health administration of these populations to international agencies and NGOs. This gives MSF the advantage of "extra-territoriality". It has the margin for manoeuvre it needs to take rapid control of all the stages in the response to an epidemic, including setting up and exploiting a surveillance system for the on-going collection of health data, epidemic investigation (with diagnosis confirmation, when necessary using biological tests) and the introduction of measures for reducing the number of infections and mortality (early detection and treatment of cases, isolation and immunisation and vector control).

In open settings, however, each of these stages must, in theory, be authorised by the host government, meaning MSF's willingness to take control of the response to an epidemic conflicts with national prerogatives. Should we then deduce from this, as suggested by MSF-France's president in 1997 that "the freedom of action [of MSF in this type of context] is virtually nil, and the quality of aid provided is almost entirely dependent on the quality of the relations developed with the administrative authorities"?[7] Should MSF's teams see cooperation with the national politico-administrative authorities as a constraint, a tactical necessity or an objective in itself? To what extent, in what conditions and with what consequences can a government's health priorities concord with those set by a humanitarian medical actor such as MSF in the management of an epidemic?

This chapter examines these issues by drawing on three specific periods in the history of MSF-Holland's and MSF-France's actions in the northern Nigerian states of Kano and Katsina (1996 to 2001, 2005, 2009). However, it is not our intention to imply that the entire history of the organisation's actions in Nigeria can be summed up in these three episodes. MSF-Holland, for example, whose misadventures in Kano we will be recounting, began responding to medical emergencies in other north Nigerian states as early as 2005. It also ran an HIV treatment programme in Lagos for several years. MSF-France, whose operations in Katsina will be described in this chapter, opened a traumatology centre in 2004 in Port Harcourt in the Niger Delta in a situation of armed conflict and, in 2008, it began an obstetrics programme in the state of Jigawa, followed in 2010 by programmes to treat malnutrition. So this chapter tells only part of the story: MSF's attempts to respond to epidemics in states where negotiations proved to be particularly complex.

Management and Perpetuation of Epidemics

Following in the wake of the 1978 Alma-Alta conference and the 1987 Bamako Initiative, the decentralisation of Nigerian health services was part of a much broader politico-administrative decentralisation that led to a series of changes in the way the country was divided up and administered. From twelve federal states in 1967, the number increased to twenty-one in 1988 and to thirty-six in 1996, with each state required to work alongside local governments (Local Government Areas, established in 1976), which were allocated a budget and run by a Local Government Council. The number of these Local Government Areas (LGAs) rose from 310 in 1989 to 774 in 1999.

This constant fragmentation has fostered competition and tensions between the different bodies, especially as the LGAs, "rather than representing a coherent community [could constitute] a zone of confrontation between factions associated in an arbitrary manner and opposing "majorities" and "minorities", chiefdoms, diverse clientele and activist groups".[8] Competition between local, federal and national health services has been particularly apparent in two crucial areas for the response to epidemics: immunisation and epidemiological surveillance.

In 1990, responsibility for primary healthcare was officially delegated to the LGAs and vaccine procurement was decentralised. This led to a drastic reduction in their availability, as the LGAs neglected to budget for them. Immunisation coverage, which had improved considerably as a result of the proactive policy implemented by Babangida's military regime (1985 to 1993) embodied by Professor Olikoye Ransome Kuti, his health minister, known in Nigeria as "the father of primary healthcare", began a relentless decline. From 1996 to 2005, the National Programme of Immunisation (NPI), which channelled the huge resources provided by the Global Polio Eradication Initiative Campaign (100 million dollars in 2006),[9] was headed by Dr Awosika, a personal friend of President Obasanjo's wife. The Nigerian media attacked her probity[10] and in December 2005, under pressure from donors, she was forced to resign. But she left a sorry legacy: national coverage for full immunisation of children under the age of one was less than 13%[11] despite "Nigeria's immunisation programme [being] by far the most expensive among developing countries around the world".[12] Called upon by donors to "restore Nigeria's dignity and honour in the international public health arena",[13] the country attempted new reforms. From 2006, initiatives financed by international donors were launched to boost primary healthcare and routine immunisation, particularly in the north of Nigeria where the situation was catastrophic. In 2005, the coverage rate in northern states for the full immunisation of children was only 4%. Three years later, it had still only reached 6% and outbreaks of measles were commonplace.

As for epidemiological surveillance, this has been hampered by an uncoordinated accumulation of public and private stakeholders. The federal Health Ministry admitted that "the existing health information system in Nigeria is characterised by extensive duplication of data collection, entry and analysis (no fewer than fifty data forms are in use at the federal level alone); multiple data pathways; lack of standard case definitions; lack of clarity with regards to data submission and responsibilities [...]".[14] Sentinel sites, the infectious disease notification system set up by the WHO, data collected from hospitals, health centres and epidemiology units, demographic statistics, NPI data and information gathered for international partners combined to create a silent cacophony. Health alerts rarely come through official channels, usually arriving too late via the press or individuals acting "unofficially", such as this employee of the WHO, between 1996 and 2009, who provided MSF with off the record health data, trusting the organisation to ensure "this data [... would] be used to further the A-C-T-I-O-N".[15]

To complicate things further, Nigeria has a system of fiscal federalism that fosters opaque management of public funds. The large majority of federal funding allocations destined for the country's other two administrative levels are paid into a "Local and State Joint Account" to be shared between the states and Local Government Areas. This constitutional provision encourages clientelist relations, as the two levels are only accountable to each other, and "horror stories"[16] often circulate about the misappropriation of funds. In 1996, federal allocations had just been paid to the Kaduna LGA in northern Nigeria to fund its response to the meningitis epidemic. When governmental medical personnel came to ask for the means to contain the increasing number of cases being registered in the villages, the head of the medical unit responded by saying that there were neither vaccines nor drugs. Instead, he advised them to give the villagers "water injections in place of vaccines for psychological satisfaction".[17]

The absence of control, coordination and efficient management has created cracks in the system that allow interests totally unrelated to public health to take hold with an impunity that grew during the periods of disorganisation generated by the epidemics in Nigeria. MSF was a direct witness to this during a meningitis epidemic in Niger in April 1995 when its teams attempted to use part of a batch of 88,000 vaccines given to the Nigerian Programme of Immunisation the previous month by the Nigerian government and the state of Sokoto. The teams rapidly encountered problems with dilution and found filaments in the vaccines, so they refused to use them. Alerted by MSF, Laboratoires Mérieux, whose name featured on the vaccines, carried out an analysis. The vaccines turned out to be fakes, containing no traces of active products. According to MSF's estimations, they had been administered to 60,000 people. Mérieux filed a counterfeit suit, followed by an international letter rogatory, but legal proceedings rapidly ground to a halt.[18]

In 1996, MSF was witness to a public scandal that is still being talked about fifteen years on. At the infectious diseases hospital in

Kano where its team was based during the meningitis epidemic, Pfizer laboratories was testing a toxic drug called Trovan on children.[19] Four years later, *The Washington Post* published an article entitled, "As drug testing spreads, profits and lives hang in the balance".[20] The article, backed up by testimony from MSF's teams, revealed the conditions in which these tests had been conducted. It accused Pfizer of using the meningitis epidemic as an opportunity for carrying out large-scale clinical testing without adequate controls, monopolising the already overstretched Nigerian medical staff and neglecting to obtain the informed consent of families too distressed to make a rational decision. At a national investigation committee set up in 2001, MSF relayed the testimony of parents who complained of not having being told they were participating in research. These families, followed by the government of Kano, filed a lawsuit against Pfizer. The case was finally settled out of court in 2009 when the pharmaceutical company agreed to pay 35 million dollars to the families of the children involved in the trials and 30 million dollars to the state of Kano, despite suspicions of complaisance on the part of the state for having authorised Pfizer to carry out the trials. According to a number of observers, some Kano government representatives still hold a grudge against MSF for its role in bringing the scandal to light. Still in government or in other positions of influence, they are thought to have encouraged the Kano health authorities to shun the organisation.

This overview of the context in which MSF was working between 1996 and 2009 shows that it would be unrealistic to rely on the existing system to manage an epidemic with the sole aim of caring for those threatened by it. On the contrary, intervening in such a context implies working outside the system and seeking allies.

Reform from Within

MSF-Holland was the first to pursue the organisation's objectives in the north of Nigeria, launching an emergency preparedness and epidemic response project which ran from 1997 to 2001.

The initial operational strategy was defined by members of the same team that had coordinated MSF's action during the major meningitis epidemic in 1996, followed later that year by a measles and cholera epidemic. It analysed the situation as follows: "The federal State has no motivation whatsoever to manage epidemics [...] unless they become a political issue. The regime (Sani Abacha's military regime) is not willing to face the international consequences of declaring an epidemic or the political embarrassment of admitting it can't control the situation [...]". The team also recommended that MSF carry out targeted projects of limited scope and avoid spreading its resources too thinly. They viewed cooperation with the authorities as a necessary evil: "As a partner in this endeavour, the Ministry of Health can't always be avoided, but it is not recommended".[21]

When the project was first launched in 1997, MSF's team worked closely with UNICEF and the WHO to train federal and state Health Ministry staff and Nigerian Red Cross personnel in epidemiological surveillance and the treatment of infectious diseases. In 1997, MSF trained forty people from the Ministry of Health in four states and in 1998 it trained 216 in ten states, only to conclude that the programme had had "no significant impact on the ability of the States to respond to epidemics".[22]

From 1999, the political situation in the north of Nigeria made it extremely difficult for MSF to pursue its objectives. After thirteen years of military government, Olusegun Obasanjo was elected president of Nigeria and dislodged the representatives of the northern states from the federal political arena. Between 1999 and 2007, these representatives seized every opportunity to assert their identity, threatened by a regime accused of favouring the interests of one region (the south), one ethnic group (the Yoruba) and one religion (Christianity). Control over public health initiatives became the object of a power struggle between the federal state and the states in the north, with MSF caught up in the middle.

In 1999, the MSF programme focused on Kano and set up a "sentinel surveillance system", which had only just been put in place when a cholera epidemic broke out. Alerted by MSF's teams, the Kano and federal health ministries denied the appearance of cholera for four whole weeks, refuting the results of laboratory analyses obtained by the organisation. They did not want to be accused of spoiling the FIFA (International Federation of Association Football) under-20s competition which Nigeria was hosting that April. MSF's reaction was to bypass the system and go to the press. In doing so, it deliberately ignored a warning made by the government in 1996 in a thank-you letter sent by the federal Ministry of Health to MSF's head of mission after the meningitis campaign: "I have been requested to advise you not to publish any data on these epidemics without the permission of the federal Ministry of Health and would ask you not to issue any statements on these epidemics that may cause embarrassment to the Federal Government of Nigeria".

That same year, while helping the teams at Kano hospital to manage a sharp increase in the number of measles cases, MSF discovered that expired vaccines were being used on the children's ward.

In April 2000, MSF's teams diagnosed a case of yellow fever in Kano, confirmed by a test that had been carried out in a Nigerian laboratory. The risk of a yellow fever epidemic had been identified when the programme was first opened, as the last epidemic dated back to 1986 and there had been no mass vaccination campaign since. Yet there is no treatment for yellow fever and the case fatality rate can exceed 50%. MSF contacted the Kano Health Ministry offering to carry out a vaccination campaign to prevent the epidemic from spreading, in line with WHO recommendations. The ministry at first accepted before retracting and refuting the validity of the diagnosis. The head of mission turned to the religious authorities of Kano, the WHO and the federal government for support in convincing the health authorities, but to no avail. For a while, absurdly contradictory positions coexisted: MSF's teams were training Kano's medical personnel in yellow fever vaccination, while their supervisory ministry, in spite of the alert, refused to contemplate such an operation. But the expected epidemic did not occur. The head of mission summed up: "The health commissioner took a huge gamble with the health of his people and, as things turned out, he won".[23]

After two years of virtually fruitless cooperation, a cholera epidemic and the threat of a yellow fever epidemic treated with nonchalance by the health authorities, in 2001 MSF's frustration came to a head during the measles epidemic in Kano. The stonewalling, delays and negligence it was to encounter dramatically illustrated the deep-rooted problems in a system that MSF had spent five unsuccessful years trying to change. At the beginning of 2001, Kano's main public hospital was overwhelmed by a measles epidemic. By March, the surveillance system operated jointly by MSF and the Kano Health Ministry reported more than 9,000 cases in just four weeks, more than ten times as many as the previous year at the same period. The Kano Health Ministry's attempts to carry out a vaccination campaign were immediately complicated by its fraught relations with Dr Awosika, director of the

National Programme of Immunisation (NPI), who requisitioned the medical and logistical equipment needed for the campaign in order to run the National Polio Immunisation Days.

For several weeks, the federal Health Ministry refused entry to the imported drugs which MSF had ordered; it was only after the governor intervened in March that they were eventually authorised. In April it took MSF several weeks of negotiations to obtain permission from the Kano Health Ministry to set up a tent in the grounds of the hospital, despite the fact that the hospital, overwhelmed by the influx of measles cases, had stopped admitting new patients several weeks earlier. MSF's teams finally managed to take charge of the coordination of treatment in the hospital, working alongside governmental staff. The epidemic was at its height, but MSF struggled to coordinate an unmotivated care team, some of whom decided to go on strike. In May, when the measles fatality rate in the hospital exceeded 25%, MSF asked the health commissioner for permission to carry out an awareness-raising campaign to encourage parents to bring their children to hospital as early as possible. He refused, and proceeded to make a public statement in which he played down the health problem.

This was the last straw. MSF decided to confront the Kano health authorities with what it saw as a repeated neglect of their responsibilities and sent a letter terminating its intervention to the Health Ministry, copied to the National Programme of Immunisation, the federal Health Ministry, the religious authorities of Kano, the WHO and international funding agencies. The letter contained a series of criticisms and protestations about the attitude of the health authorities, describing five years of difficult cooperation and bitterly concluding that there was a "lack of political commitment and transparency", and that "political interests [took] precedence over humanitarian interests, resulting in a senseless loss of human life". The organisation expressed its "disappointment" in the lack of cooperation on the part of the Kano authorities, which had made no changes despite "numerous discussions with MSF", and their lack of interest in the training delivered by MSF. The letter was followed by a diplomatic visit to each of its recipients. The main parties concerned gave MSF a good-natured welcome. The Kano health minister thanked MSF for everything it had done and said she would invite the organisation back soon, the federal health minister promised to look into the problems in Kano and the WHO advised patience. This is how MSF's operational experience in Kano came to an end.

From 1997 to 2001, MSF's teams were prisoners of their cooperation with the health authorities at a time when, in fact, they needed
considerable operational latitude. The failure of MSF's objectives, at
first masked by the consensual nature of its initial collaborations and
training programmes, was eventually confirmed by its inability to take
action or convince the authorities, and sometimes even the state medical personnel, of the need to take action or, in other words, to change
their attitude and their priorities.

In the years that followed, MSF published articles denouncing the
Kano authorities' lack of political commitment towards health issues,[24]
but they found little resonance in Nigerian public debate.

Voluntary Capitulation

In 2005, MSF's French section ran a malnutrition treatment programme for several months during a measles epidemic affecting the
state of Adamawa in the north east zone of Nigeria. Then in June
2005, alerted by MSF's mission in Maradi in Niger to the increasing
number of malnourished children arriving from Katsina, the organisation decided to carry out an exploratory mission in this state bordering Kano. The situation discovered by the mission was worrying; the
people had just been hit by a measles epidemic and, as MSF knew from
experience, measles epidemics are usually followed by an increase in
the number of cases of malnutrition. To make things worse, the price
of cereals was much higher than the previous year at the same period.

After a meeting with the health authorities that included the permanent secretary for health, (second only to the health minister), it took
just a few days for MSF to obtain the authorisations it needed to open
a programme to treat severe acute malnutrition in Katsina. The permanent secretary was a close friend and the personal doctor of Umaru
Yar'Adua, the governor of Katsina and a candidate in the presidential
elections due to be held in 2007. The authorities' initial reception was
warm. Looking back, the head of mission at the time describes MSF's
first steps in Katsina as being something akin to "a honeymoon before
the wedding".

At the end of July, MSF opened a nutrition stabilisation centre in
Katsina for cases of complicated severe acute malnutrition, as well as
six outpatient centres for treating simple severe acute malnutrition,
admitting more than 600 children a week. However, as the programme

gained visibility and began attracting media attention, MSF's official contacts quickly began to show signs of concern. The stabilisation centre in Katsina was overflowing and MSF was attempting to open other centres when, in August, a *Reuters* article was published with the headline: "Child malnutrition hits thousands in Nigerian north". The article went on to say that Nigeria was not a "destitute" country like neighbouring Niger, which was facing serious food shortages, but a country with a "history of corruption and mismanagement [that had] failed to translate its oil wealth into basic services for the majority of its people". Needless to say, Katsina's authorities, who had just publicly announced that they were sending aid to Niger,[25] were furious. The permanent secretary of Katsina's Health Ministry had no intention of letting pictures of emaciated children give the impression that the state was incapable of taking care of its people and risk spoiling the start of the governor's election campaign, a campaign that he himself was supporting.

With MSF's authorisation to work in Katsina due to expire on 13 September 2005, the situation became increasingly tense. Health Ministry representatives hammered home the same message at every meeting: MSF must leave as quickly as possible and let them take over the programme. And so began a race against the clock, with the ministry pushing MSF to train as many government staff as possible in preparation for taking over the programme and MSF attempting to admit as many children as it could to persuade the ministry that it was not capable of taking charge of such a large-scale project. MSF's project coordinator commented at the time: "They still think they're going to turf us out at the end [of the agreement] on 13 September, but if we keep up admissions in the first seven LGAs, and add a few more in the new ones, by the middle of September we'll have over 2,000 people on the nutrition programme and it'll be impossible for them to take over and cope with so many patients. We'll see what happens, but we're looking to boost the programme as much as we can to have as many beneficiaries as possible (dual objective: care and pressure)".[26] As the situation escalated, the teams threatened to "go public" and at one point, after trying to convince the authorities that "without rapid and appropriate intervention 50% of the severely malnourished children [would] die",[27] even considered opening new centres without authorisation.

In the end, there was no confrontation. The authorities gave MSF a few more weeks and, by the end of September, the number of patients started to decrease. The teams began closing outpatient centres with fewer than a hundred beneficiaries. This resulted in a reduction in the number of referrals of sick children to the stabilisation centre in Katsina and, from that point on, the teams adhered strictly to patient discharge criteria. Soon they were no longer arguing for the opening of a new stabilisation centre.

After fighting to maintain its nutrition programmes in what it had perceived as a severe crisis situation, MSF's teams seemed increasingly convinced that the organisation had no further role to play when malnutrition was no longer "epidemic", but had become "endemic". In November, after a meeting between the coordination team and the team at head office, MSF began closing the programme. It briefly considered communicating publicly about the need to maintain some kind of malnutrition treatment service, but in the end left Katsina as discreetly as possible so as not to compromise its chances of returning in the future. The teams handed the activities over to the authorities, but had few illusions about what would become of them: "We knew that the government wasn't serious about taking over the activities, although we tried to convince ourselves otherwise as we were leaving. But three days after our departure, the stabilisation centre was empty and they had stopped admitting children into the outpatients programme so they could close it down by the end of January".[28] In closing the programme so hurriedly, the Health Ministry's priority was to remove all trace of MSF and its embarrassing activities before the governor of Katsina began his campaign for the 2007 presidential elections—elections that he went on to win.

MSF's action in Katsina allowed 12,000 children to be treated for malnutrition during a critical period, due to the teams' success in negotiating an additional few weeks of operation beyond the original deadline. Once the visibility of MSF's activities and the media attention they attracted became an embarrassment to the health authorities, the organisation was caught up in a battle of wills. It held its own thanks to two weighty arguments. Firstly, only MSF was capable of managing such a large number of patients and if it had been forced to abandon them from one day to the next, the authorities would have had an extremely difficult situation on their hands. Secondly, with the presidential elections looming, the authorities were more receptive to the threat of going public than usual. By making malnutrition visible, MSF was able to exert direct influence on the authorities. But, by then accepting to make it invisible again, even to itself, it gave up on regarding severe acute malnutrition as a public health problem that its know-how, innovative skills and influence could help resolve.

Public (Health) Relations

In 2006, as part of a more global strategy for improving its capacity to respond to emergencies in the north, MSF-France set up a mobile surveillance and reaction team of Nigerian doctors. This "emergency pool" soon focused on Jigawa State, where the health authorities were cooperative, and Kano and Katsina States. Designed to be simple and responsive, it was based on a network of willing participants from within the Nigerian health system. The network, developed by MSF over the course of its misadventures relayed alerts to members of the emergency pool who would then try to verify the situation on the ground, assisted by other allies who facilitated their access to field data. Between 2006 and 2008, while managing to respond to a series of medical emergencies in those states willing to cooperate—measles and malnutrition in Yobe, cholera in Borno and meningitis in Jigawa—MSF also made several attempts to respond to alerts in Katsina and Kano. The organisation was never able to obtain official authorisation to gather data or conduct surveys on measles, malnutrition and cholera alerts during this period, and so had no objective justification for the intervention proposals it took to the health authorities. Yet these same health authorities were quite willing to discuss meningitis with MSF. In 2008, its teams were thus able to vaccinate almost 100,000 people in Katsina. Although the circumstances did little to help make the operation a success (late intervention and difficulties in establishing vaccination priorities because of incoherencies in the data from the surveillance system), at least they had the assent of all the health authorities. After a visit to Katsina at the beginning of April 2008, the Nigerian coordinator of the emergency pool remarked: "I must admit that the authorities welcomed the idea of MSF taking part in the meningitis vaccination campaign. But they were against any other form of 'invasion', especially in the area of nutrition".[29]

Indeed, meningitis, which affects both children and adults, is a disease that has considerable political advantages as far as governments are concerned. Whereas cholera and measles reveal, respectively, the insalubrity of water and sanitation infrastructures and the failures of routine immunisation programmes, and malnutrition highlights the fact that the state is incapable of feeding its people, meningitis epidemics "pose little threat to governments, because in the absence of prevention measures they do not get blamed when people are affected [...]. Not only can the government not be held responsible for the scourge, it can ride to the rescue by organising mass vaccination campaigns".[30] It goes without saying that the governments of north Nigeria were even more keen to organise a response given that what would be a useful public relations exercise was to be largely sponsored by external volunteers such as MSF.

Another occasion for conducting such a public relations exercise arose in 2009 during a large-scale meningitis epidemic which saw the Spanish, Dutch and French sections working simultaneously in nine different states. MSF-France initially concentrated on Jigawa and Katsina, skirting round the intransigent Kano where it had tried in vain to obtain authorisation to intervene before deciding, after two fruitless weeks of negotiation, also to concentrate on the state of Bauchi. In four months, the sections vaccinated over 4.7 million people, with more than 1.5 million in the state of Katsina alone. Immunisation coverage was good, "relations with the authorities [were] very satisfactory and the authorities [were] satisfied with MSF's work".[31]

At first sight, the operation was thus a success; it allowed MSF's teams to take large-scale action on a major public health problem with the assent and then the congratulations of health authorities who were traditionally recalcitrant towards MSF's interventions. But what real impact did it have on the epidemics?

The polysaccharide vaccine used by MSF[32] induces a weak and transitory immunological memory of about two or three years. It has no immunogenic power in children under the age of two and only limited power in children under the age of four, and it does not eliminate carriage.[33] As early as 1996, at the end of the mass vaccination campaign run by MSF in north Nigeria, research based on observation data gathered during the campaign concluded that because it had taken place several weeks after the epidemic thresholds had been crossed, the effect had been "marginal", averting only 3.3% of cases in the state of Katsina.[34] The medical conclusions drawn from the operation therefore pleaded in favour of an increased focus on patient treatment and early and highly localised immunisation campaigns, rather than mass vaccination during an epidemic, all the more since this last strategy requires massive human and material resources that would be more useful to strengthen patient case management.

Thirteen years later, on the eve of the 2009 meningitis epidemic, the organisation was much better armed to respond effectively. It was no longer in terra incognita and its emergency pool of Nigerian doctors had increased its reaction capacity. Yet the operation was hardly an out-and-out success. A survey carried out by MSF revealed that the efforts of hundreds of its employees in vaccinating 1.5 million people in Katsina prevented the occurrence of 4.4% of cases.[35] Furthermore, the real impact of the campaign on the decline in the epidemic was as difficult to establish in 2009 as it had been in 1996, as the arrival of the rainy season in May interrupts the transmission of the bacteria.

Therefore, the speed of MSF's initial intervention in Katsina, though quite remarkable, had only a marginal impact on the effectiveness of the vaccination campaign. For to be effective, the difficulty is "being sensitive enough to react as quickly as possible, but specific enough not to launch unnecessary campaigns".[36] In other words, a vaccination campaign must be carried out very shortly after epidemic thresholds have been crossed. However, in Nigeria, organising a meningitis vaccination campaign that satisfies these criteria is an impossible task. The structural weaknesses of the surveillance systems and the time needed to organise such an operation mean that however rapidly the teams react, interventions are unavoidably late. According to the WHO's epidemic preparedness and response coordinator, the operation was essentially a response to the demands of the authorities and the population, as claiming the right conditions existed for an effective meningitis vaccination campaign in Nigeria would be pure "science fiction".[37] Furthermore, the health authorities had stressed the need to make the response appear equitable, the idea being to vaccinate as many people in as many places as possible in order to reassure the population as a whole. It was in order to satisfy this demand that in 2009 MSF's teams in Katsina agreed to vaccinate certain zones, regardless of epidemiological considerations.

In 1996, during MSF's medical symposium on infectious diseases, Dr Michel Rey, one of the experts on meningitis who helped devise the treatments the organisation uses today, remarked that: "Until now, all the mass vaccination campaigns intended to control a meningitis epidemic have been carried out after the epidemic peak. This type of action may be beneficial from a political point of view, but it is questionable from a public health standpoint".[38]

What were the "political gains" from the 2009 vaccination campaign other than public relations benefits? The Kano health authorities, who MSF hoped would relent when they saw what was being done in neighbouring states, remained impervious to argument. However, those in Katsina opened up and, in 2010, MSF's teams were occasionally invited in to support health facilities during measles and cholera epidemics. But MSF's ambitions continued to be restricted to satisfying the demands of the health authorities. It is our theory that, ultimately, MSF's setbacks with the most recalcitrant north Nigerian states imperceptibly influenced its objectives: in its desire to win over the health and political authorities, the need to act prevailed over the reasons for doing so.

The attempts to respond to epidemics in the north of Nigeria, which were as much attempts to bring to heel those in power, reveal the limits to cooperation between a humanitarian medical operator and health and political authorities. In the face of public health issues, mutual acculturation is not enough to make the divergences between these authorities and MSF disappear, as the organisation's experience in Kano has shown. Nor can their priorities be influenced by the "saving lives" argument, as seen in MSF's failed attempt in Katsina. Ultimately, the meningitis episode in 2009 shows that achieving convergence on health priorities between political authorities and MSF can be at the expense of the pertinence of its interventions and risks narrowing its operational horizons down to those of its hosts.

An alternative to this tempering of MSF's ambitions would be to develop not good relations with the authorities, but the right conditions for achieving a balance of power with them. How? Perhaps by being less predictable, and so less vulnerable, in the negotiations with the north Nigerian politico-administrative powers: by curbing its taste for action when the reasons for acting do not require it, and by taking the risk of incurring the authorities' displeasure by daring to expose, publicly if necessary, the neglected issues on which it can legitimately deploy its expertise, such as the treatment and prevention of acute malnutrition and measles.

Translated from French by Mandy Duret

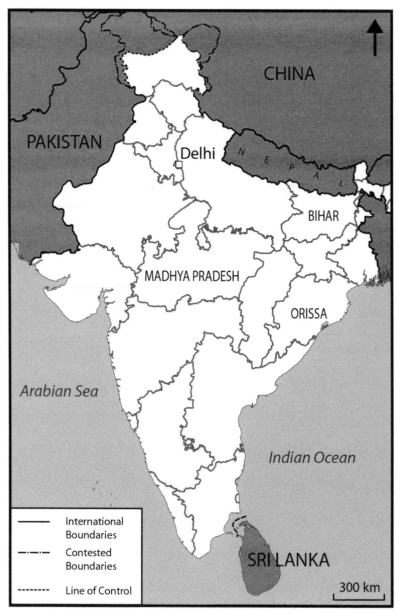

India

INDIA

THE EXPERT AND THE MILITANT

Stéphane Doyon

In 2005, MSF's work in the Maradi region of Niger proved the large-scale effectiveness of new strategies based on the use of ready-to-use therapeutic foods (RUTF)[1] for outpatient treatment of severe acute malnutrition.[2] The MSF teams treated 60,000 malnourished children in just a few months and, by the end of the treatment, almost 80% of them were cured. Results as good as these were unattainable using previous treatment protocols, which necessitated the hospitalisation of all children. In 2007, MSF and the Campaign for Access to Essential Medicines[3] set out to increase access to RUTF by promoting, in Niger for example, the development of initiatives for local production of the milk paste and also actively encouraging research and development. The opportunities for mass treatment offered by RUTF prompted MSF to become involved in regions where malnutrition was endemic and to strive to bring about reforms to national and international nutrition policies.

India, with around 40% of the world's severely malnourished children,[4] gives MSF the opportunity to put its political and operational ambitions into practice, especially as malnutrition is not a taboo subject in the subcontinent. During his speech marking the 60th anniversary of Indian independence in 2007, the Prime Minister Manmohan Singh stated that: "The problem of malnutrition is a national shame. I appeal to the nation to do the utmost to eradicate malnutrition within five years".[5]

The rate of malnutrition in India remains constant, or may even be increasing, an embarrassment to the government on two levels. First, because it highlights the failure of national initiatives, such as the Integrated Child Development Services programme set up in 1975 and designed to provide children under six with ready-made meals at community health centres known as *Anganwadis*. Second, it is proof that India's economic growth has failed to reduce malnutrition, as a number of national and international observers have pointed out. The Indian Association of Paediatricians commented that, "despite improvements in economy, health sector, literacy, and health and nutritional indicators, the prevalence of severe acute malnutrition [as defined by WHO norms] is still unacceptably rife, particularly among children under three years old".[6] The most recent national surveys, conducted in 2005–6,[7] show that "infant malnutrition is increasing despite the economic boom" in India, as highlighted by an Indian journalist who specialises in development issues.[8] For example, in Haryana, one of the subcontinent's most prosperous states, the rate of chronic child malnutrition among under three-year-olds rose from 34.4% in 1998–99 to 41.9% in 2005–06, with acute cases rising from 5.3% to 16.7% during the same period. The international press pushed the point home: "The results [of the 2006 national survey] provide a shocking illustration of how India's recent economic boom, while enriching the social elite and the middle classes, has failed to benefit almost half of its 1.1 billion people",[9] wrote a *Times* journalist in 2006 in an article with the provocative heading "Indian children suffer more malnutrition than in Ethiopia".

For those called on by the prime minister to tackle malnutrition, Right to Food campaign in India[10] occupies a special place. An initiative driven by campaigners, trade unions, people's movements, NGOs, experts and human rights organisations, it was established in 2001 after the Indian Supreme Court was petitioned to require the government to use its food stocks to combat the food shortages threatening the population. Since then, the Supreme Court, acting on information provided by Indian civil society, issues interim court orders which carry the force of law, enjoining the government to protect the right to food, primarily through guaranteeing access to national programmes such as school canteens, food distributions and work for food programmes.

According to Right to Food, malnutrition has to be examined from all angles: the deepening agrarian crisis, public policies that ignore children, gender inequality, the dismantlement of the public distribution system, the caste system, as well as the growing influence of commercial forces in the manufacture of products for infants, genetically modified seeds and experiments in biotechnology. Its members organise demonstrations, publish scientific analyses and draft proposals for legislation to alter the legal framework and content of national social and food programmes. As some members hold official positions, their opinions are more likely to influence the process of changing India's policies and laws. For instance, Biraj Patnaik, one of the key persons of Right to Food, is principal adviser to the Commissioners of the Supreme Court on the right to food.

Right to Food calls on a whole range of strategies to exert pressure, including legal activism, raising awareness and protest. It also consults and works with the state, which it sees as having a specific role to play in as much as it is responsible for ensuring the food and nutritional security of the Indian people through improving the quality of its services. Therefore, neither the Indian state nor Right to Food will allow the issue of malnutrition to be addressed by foreign aid organisations, accused of defending their own interests to the detriment of the common interest. In 2003, India banned food aid donations from US NGOs because it considered the enriched flour distributed liable to be contaminated by genetic modification, and thus unfit for human consumption.[11] Indian civil society organisations took this as proof that this type of overseas aid "was nothing but a prelude to opening the doors for commercial dumping of [genetically modified] foods by the US multinationals that are unable to find markets in Europe".[12]

Differing Ideas About Malnutrition

MSF and Right to Food would appear to have a common enemy in malnutrition; however, each organisation perceives different realities and different solutions, as was immediately apparent when they first met in 2008. For MSF, tackling a public health issue of this kind demands first and foremost providing an answer to the medical emer-

gency, in this case acute malnutrition, where the body starts to con-
sume its own tissue in order to find the energy and nutrients it needs to
survive. However, this is not a concept favoured in India, where malnutrition is seen as a problem that slows down children's development
and reveals that their food needs are not being met. Put another way,
where MSF sees malnutrition as a potentially fatal condition that has
to be combated through the use of appropriate treatment, Right to
Food perceives it primarily as a signifier of social injustice that entitles
its victims to receive assistance from the state. These diverging concepts underscore the differences in the way to finding priority solutions
to malnutrition.

The development of an outpatient nutrition rehabilitation system
had been under debate at MSF ever since the first experiments in Niger
in 2002, as it required a shift in the organisation's practices and
assumptions.[13] Handing over most of the responsibility for administering nutritional treatment to the children's mothers meant giving up
close monitoring of a child's medical condition, as under previous protocols and during the hospitalisation they necessitated. Paradoxically,
the medicalisation of malnutrition entailed a degree of demedicalisa-
tion in the way that MSF worked, rendered acceptable in terms of
medical effectiveness by the introduction of RUTF. Switching to the use
of ready-to-eat pastes meant no more careful preparation of water- and
milk-based therapeutic rations under conditions of strict hygiene, and
that nursing care was no longer as necessary in treating children. In
fact, no matter how severe the malnutrition, providing that the child
wants to eat, s/he can be given individual milk paste sachets and
allowed to go home. Treatment dosages are very simple to follow and
a weekly check-up on the weight curve is quite sufficient.

However, whereas MSF saw RUTF as a chance to simplify the distribution, administration and use of nutritional treatments, essential if
medical responsibility was to be delegated to the families of malnourished children, Right to Food perceived a risk of exacerbating poverty
and social demobilisation. Its members felt that the response to the issue
of malnutrition had to include increasing points of contact between
marginalised groups—women, lower castes—and the rest of society.
Over four million Indian women[14] are employed preparing meals for
children, a task that offers great scope for social interaction.

Plumpy'nut, the therapeutic food used by MSF in most of its programmes, is a commercial product made overseas and patented in a
number of countries.[15] Some members of Right to Food viewed it as a

Trojan horse for the very international food industry that the campaign is committed to fighting against.[16] In April 2008, its members staged a protest during a meeting organised in India by GAIN (Global Alliance for Improved Nutrition), an international foundation linked to private business whose stated aim is to combat malnutrition by making sure that suitable products are available on the market. During the meeting, Right to Food members demanded that GAIN "spare India from its strategy that seeks to build promising markets for multinationals and the food industry [such as] Unilever, Cargill, Danone and Wockhardt" and congratulated the government for not "succumbing to the biscuit manufacturers' lobbies and resisting their attempts to replace distributed hot meals [as part of the government nutritional programmes]".[17]

The most vocal and radical wing of Right to Food against the commercialisation of food and the industry's conflict of interest is the BPNI (Breastfeeding Promotion Network in India), which grew from the movement to fight the sales strategies used by Nestlé in Africa during the 1970s to promote its baby formula products. The coordinator of the world's largest network for the promotion of breastfeeding, Dr Gupta, accused MSF of the "legitimisation of commercial products for feeding young children [...] by creating a simplistic solution for child malnutrition".[18] Dr Gupta was all the more suspicious because of MSF's stated aim of using RUTF derivatives to prevent malnutrition, as expressed in its public documents and at international scientific conferences. He declared that: "The story of one success in an emergency situation [in Niger] is quickly being translated into a mainstream intervention for preventing and treating severe child malnutrition. [...]. Once we start using RUFs [ready to use foods] as a preventive strategy, as is being voiced by these international agencies, child nutrition turns into a big market".[19]

It is against this background that three different approaches were set in motion by three different organisations, all apparently inspired by the same goal of treating severe acute malnutrition in India. These were direct and discreet action, led by MSF-Spain; the alliance with Right to Food, incarnated by the Access Campaign; and the strategy of the widespread fait accompli, as adopted by UNICEF from 2008.

Take Action and Prescribe

In August of 2007, Bihar State was hit by flooding and MSF-Spain set up a two-month mobile consultation service in Dharbanga district. During this period, the MSF teams identified a large number of malnourished children and treated around 1,000 of them with Plumpy'nut. MSF closed its programme once the floods abated, but decided to carry out a nutritional survey in the area. Their suspicions were confirmed: 20% of children were suffering from acute malnutrition, and almost 5% were severely malnourished,[20] sufficient according to established international standards to constitute an emergency situation. A food security survey conducted by MSF found that malnutrition "is not episodic and related to the 2007 floods, but is an endemic, long-term problem".[21]

So MSF decided to set up a programme in Dharbanga district. In geographical terms, the choice stemmed from the gravity of the nutritional and health situation seen to affect the population and to which no local responses were forthcoming. Being directly confronted with this state of affairs led MSF-Spain to decide to take action on the question of malnutrition, and in 2008 it began talks at the local level. In the words of the programme manager: "This project was not driven by a political agenda set by the organisation's head offices. It started in the field [...]. We still don't know where it will lead, but we have to accept an element of trial-and-error and uncertainty. The main thing today is to be able to save these children's lives".[22] A remote area with very few social and medical facilities, it is regularly affected by widespread flooding during the monsoon season, causing people to flee their homes and making access extremely difficult. Although such precarious conditions were sufficient to justify action, they also represented obstacles, potentially undermining MSF in achieving its goal of substantiating the programme's results, which required ongoing monitoring of patients, including in their own homes, in order to be able to establish the "scientific proof" that would help to convince Indian public opinion.

MSF-Spain was not primarily seeking to prove the effectiveness of its strategy, or to transform the way that nutritionally fragile children were cared for at the national level; it sought simply to act immediately and locally. The modesty of its aims was motivated by the desire to avoid repeating its recent experiences with the treatment of visceral leishmaniasis, another pathology endemic to India with 80–90% of known sufferers in Bihar State. Aiming to bring about a change in the national treatment protocol, MSF had worked very closely with the Health Ministry and an Indian research institute, as well as conducting lengthy and elaborate negotiations with local and national authorities before finally arriving at the first phase: authorisation to use the treatment of its own choosing in its programmes. MSF felt, as it said publicly, that all this had taken too much time: "After a drawn-out year-long bureaucratic process, MSF-Spain has started to receive and treat patients suffering from visceral leishmaniasis".[23] So the Spanish section set out to treat malnutrition immediately and swiftly, avoiding or ignoring as far as possible the procedural straitjacket that it had encountered when attempting to alter nationwide practices in the treatment of leishmaniasis. Initially seeking a low profile for its activities, the organisation hoped that in due course its programme results would speak for themselves and enable it to lobby in favour of changes to malnutrition treatment in India.

On the other hand, the Access Campaign which supported MSF-France's objective of starting a nutrition project in India as of 2007, was determined right from the start to play a part in reshaping national practices and policies: "The idea was to set up a pilot programme to show that this was a do-able and effective way of treating severe acute malnutrition and [...] to play a part in spreading the word about this type of treatment across the country, inciting civil society, intellectual and political leaders to take up the cause".[24] The MSF section decided to turn to the Access Campaign's Indian office, set up in 2005 to lobby for a legal and judicial framework in favour of domestic production of low-cost generic drugs and working hand-in-hand with other civil society organisations across India. One key person of the Access Campaign India, and with close ties to Right to Food, forecast the failure of a project parachuted in from outside, and advised that the section should work closely with Indian civil society and the government to seek an Indian solution to malnutrition. Yet, this person accepted to be part of an MSF evaluation team with two ardent proponents of the widespread use of RUTF, which visited a district in Orissa State during July 2008. A rapid examination of children based on an evaluation of their brachial perimeters revealed that one in ten was suffering from severe acute malnutrition,[25] a reality that the representative of the Access Campaign India had never previously encountered. Striving to find treatment solutions, the team discovered that the local government programme canteens had no food to offer. It also found that local stores only stocked what one team-member dubbed "compassion treatments" for malnutrition, meaning foods whose composition failed to meet the specific needs of malnourished children. By the end of their evaluation, the three members of the team were in agreement: government and market were both unable to offer solutions to the problem of severe acute malnutrition, but there was a network of local community organisations that a potential treatment mechanism could work with.

In August of 2008, a few weeks after the evaluation team's visit, floods once again struck India. The prime minister declared a national disaster and appealed for international assistance. MSF-France stepped in to provide primary healthcare to people living in one of the coastal areas of Orissa, and began the lengthy process of negotiating with local authorities to set up a nutrition programme.

At the same time, the dialogue between MSF and Right to Food campaigners was progressing with every meeting, facilitated by the members of the Access Campaign India as go-between, and regular visits from the Paris-based Access Campaign representative. Despite their initial differences of opinion, the people involved had confidence in MSF. They knew about its battles with the pharmaceutical industry on ensuring access to generics, and they were also increasingly sensitive to the need to develop a curative approach in the face of the eight million Indian children suffering from severe acute malnutrition. This awareness echoed the plea issued by the Indian Association of Paediatricians for the adoption of an outpatient care model: "India only has 900,000 hospital beds. It is therefore impossible from an operational point of view to admit all these [malnourished] children, which makes home-based treatment strategies an inevitable alternative".[26]

In December 2008, Right to Food representatives met with MSF to debate the issue of care in India for cases of acute malnutrition. Participants were Right to Food members most closely involved in nutrition issues, and a doctor from the National Institute of Nutrition was invited to offer a counterweight to MSF's scientific expertise and discuss the possibility of drawing up joint documents on relevant experiences. Once again, the talks foundered on the question of treatment: for Right to Food, there could be no question of accepting imports of RUTF. MSF thought that it was moving in the right direction when it announced that local production would soon come on stream, working with companies located in India, such as CIPLA and Compact,[27] and with whom it was already in negotiation. But the campaigners were adamant that commercial interests had no place in the production of a common good: they wished to support an economic model with a community-based, cooperative or public structure, preferably on a small scale. The product would have to bend to this imperative, not the other way around. The MSF position was that centralised, industrial production of RUTF would offer the best quality guarantees—product standardisation and packaging and controlled hygiene conditions—but the campaigners maintained that, because of the size of the subcontinent, it was better to risk recurrent localised quality problems than an industrial incident affecting the only production line.

MSF undertook to encourage production initiatives of the type supported by Right to Food. However, it also stated that it would use imported products in the treatment of malnutrition, because "the priority is to treat the children and if their treatment is not to be delayed we have to use whatever therapeutic products are available; it will take a long time to agree on a new local formula".[28] Approval was granted at the end of the meeting. Mindful of the imperative to do something in the face of a lamentably persistent problem, the campaigners agreed that MSF could start nutritional campaigns using imported RUTF, so long as it had no implications for the state-run programme, and they called on the organisation to come forward with scientific proof that its recommended strategies could be adapted to the context of Indian malnutrition.

Yet, even while MSF-France and MSF-Spain were in negotiations on opening their respective projects in Bihar and Orissa, the whole situation changed as a consequence of a more aggressive strategy adopted by UNICEF.

A Medical Coup d'État

UNICEF had been running a programme to combat severe malnutrition in Madhya Pradesh since 2006. It was a hybrid programme combining WHO-designed norms for detection and treatment of severe acute malnutrition and Indian practices, which differed primarily in terms of the criteria used to identify malnutrition. The programme ran Nutrition Rehabilitation Centres which offered fifteen-day in-patient care to children who were malnourished by Indian standards, i.e. chronically malnourished, and below the norm for their weight/height, as well as children who were severely emaciated. The Madhya Pradesh health authorities were amenable to UNICEF's innovation, which was to medicalise malnutrition treatment, and they helped to expand the programme; by the end of 2008, there were 182 Nutrition Rehabilitation Centres in Madhya Pradesh State.

However, for new UNICEF chief nutritional advisor Victor Aguayo, nutrition advisor to the UN in Niger in 2005 and who arrived in India in 2008, the model was overly restrictive: it required hospitalising a large number of children who could be treated as out-patients; it failed to offer a suitable solution to children suffering from chronic malnutrition; and the production of the foods was not standardised and was based on foodstuffs purchased locally and therefore not fortified with the vitamins and minerals essential to the children's recovery. His observations were backed by two international nutrition experts invited by UNICEF to report on its programme. UNICEF then decided to modify its programme protocols by introducing imported products whose quality it could vouch for. Its representatives decided to override the objections to the use of imported industrial RUTF raised by Right to Food. As became apparent during different discussions between MSF and UNICEF managers in 2008, UNICEF, having witnessed Right to Food's outspoken intervention at the meeting held by the Global Alliance for Improved Nutrition (GAIN), considered the civil society alliance to be a radical movement whose influence was restricted by their ideological heterogeneity. UNICEF therefore decided to restrict itself to dealing with state representatives alone, using an imperious argument as a justification for its reforms. The UNICEF representative in Madhya Pradesh declared: "RUTF has been a real revolution. India simply cannot say no to its use".[29]

Ironically, it was Right to Food that provided UNICEF with the opportunity to implement its reform. As campaigning got underway for the Madhya Pradesh legislative elections, to be held at the end of 2008, Right to Food's local section tried to push malnutrition onto the agenda. The state was known to be the most affected by severe malnutrition, with an estimated 1.26 million children afflicted each year,[30] and that year it was also suffering from drought. The campaigners blamed the "Madhya Pradesh government [which] seems deaf to all news about the scourge of hunger across its state [and] refuses constantly to recognise what's going on, saying that malnutrition is not the real reason for these children's deaths".[31] The media took up the story, backed by hard-hitting pictures taken in the UNICEF-supported government nutrition centres.

UNICEF grasped this opportunity to suggest a face-saving solution to the government, embarrassed by Right to Food's statements: authorise treatment strategies using Plumpy'nut, which promised fast and effective results. Faced with a health and electoral emergency, the Madhya Pradesh government approved the initiative without, however, making it official. In August 2008, use of Plumpy'nut was introduced at nutrition centres in two districts where the media had reported a great many deaths of children. Soon afterwards, flooding in Bihar gave UNICEF further grounds for taking action and it introduced Plumpy'nut there as well.

However, in October 2008, Right to Food members in Madhya Pradesh found out that UNICEF was handing out sachets of the imported food, Plumpy'nut, to children without federal government authorisation or prior consultation, and in breach of the Supreme Court's 2004 ban on the use of centrally procured commercial foods in national food programmes.

An emergency meeting attended by UNICEF and Right to Food was called in Madhya Pradesh. The principal adviser on the right to food to the Supreme Court, Biraj Patnaik, who had helped MSF nationally and internationally in highlighting malnutrition issues, tried to intercede in favour of expanding malnutrition treatments to embrace new approaches, while requiring them to be adapted to suit the Indian context. But the campaigners were highly suspicious of UNICEF: the organisation was accused of having violated the principles of national sovereignty by importing Plumpy'nut and setting up a protocol new to India without consulting the national authorities. Its ties with GAIN encouraged the idea that it was seeking primarily to open up a market for food multinationals. As provided for under the Indian constitution, Right to Food initiated a procedure requesting information from the government and demanding an investigation into how RUTF was introduced and the Indian state's responsibility in the process.

In February 2009, the ministry responsible for approving UNICEF's activity plan asked it to withdraw RUTF from its budget since the government did not allow them. The UN agency's programmes were cut off from their supplies. At the same time, apparently alerted by the more radical elements of the BPNI, a member of the national parliament put a question to the minister of health: "Is the Minister aware that UNICEF and MSF have imported industrial nutrition foods without government approval?"[32] Challenged in public to make a show of force, the Indian government ordered UNICEF to explain itself. The UN agency offered as defence the acute necessity for emergency action after the floods in Bihar and the drought in Madhya Pradesh. In a letter sent in May 2009, the minister of health reminded the agency that it was bound to obey national laws and that, in particular, it had to respect national sovereignty on nutrition and emergency response. The government further demanded not only that use of RUTF cease, but that remaining stocks be shipped out of the country and a programme of equal value be made as payment.

This dramatic turn of events had immediate consequences for MSF-France. Negotiations with the Orissa State government, which had been dragging on for several months, collapsed. The local authorities had no intention of stepping out of line with the federal government and suggested that MSF try and sort the problem out in Delhi. After a full year of talks, which had already lasted far too long in the minds of most head office desk managers, MSF decided to pull its team out and to abandon its project.

However, MSF-Spain did manage to sign an agreement with the Dharbanga district health authorities to start a project in early 2009. Admittedly, its initial scope was limited to treating severe acute malnutrition with RUTF, with no provisions for conducting research. The Spanish section had resolved to focus on setting up a local agreement so that it could start providing treatment as quickly as possible. Shielded by the discreet nature of its activities, the modesty of its stated aims, the remote area where its work was restricted to, as well as an unvoiced "live and let live" agreement with Right to Food, the Spanish section's programme went ahead unaffected by the turmoil surrounding UNICEF.

Operational Failure, Public Health Success

The Plumpy'nut controversy might have led to a halt to UNICEF's nutrition programmes, but it also triggered a national debate and considerable domestic media coverage on the question of how to "Indianise" treatment for severe malnutrition. MSF continued to play a part in the debate, alongside the All India Institute of Medical Sciences, the Indian Association of Paediatricians, Right to Food and various government representatives. In order to cut short arguments about the danger of the links between the product and the food industry, RUTF were renamed Medical Nutrition Therapies (MNT). During a consensus-building meeting held in November 2009, the Madhya Pradesh health commissioner, one of the people driving treatment for severe malnutrition in the state, presented the results of the programme set up with UNICEF. The results showed that over 33,000 children had been treated during the period 2006 to 2008, and that the use of fortified milk pastes was effective. Ironically, therefore, the very first discussion on experiences in India concerned a programme whose clandestine nature had been denounced by Right to Food and was now defended by the very people who had worked to stymie UNICEF—the Madhya Pradesh section of Right to Food.

The report on the meeting, published in the Indian Paediatrics[33] journal, recommended that consideration be given to treating malnutrition with "medical nutrition therapies", provided that said treatments were produced in India and the protocols examined by national experts. The editorial to the journal declares that: "Philosophical differences are evident regarding the choice of interventions to be adopted in the community. One view favours the sole adoption of the preventive and promotive aspects (ensuring basic nutrition and health care for all infants and children, especially promotion of breast feeding and appropriate complementary feeding) with no special emphasis on active detection and nutritional therapy of SAM children. [...]. We firmly believe that public health interventions for SAM must simultaneously focus on preventive and promotive aspects, and therapeutic interventions in the community".[34]

So "Indianisation" of treatment for malnutrition is underway, its pace dictated by the speed that consensus can be reached between activists, government representatives, scientists and invited experts, a group that includes MSF. There is now unanimity about the necessity of providing treatment for severe acute malnutrition in India, but a lot of ground still needs to be covered before malnutrition ceases to be a "national shame" and becomes a controlled public health issue. First, national nutrition stakeholders insist that anthropometric criteria for the identification of malnutrition have to be adapted to the Indian context. They want to ensure that thin children are not required to submit to international corpulence standards, and that the result will genuinely focus on reducing mortality and the consequences associated with the pathology. Working in collaboration with Indian research bodies, the health and family welfare ministries have launched initiatives to test and compare community-based treatment models that could be incorporated within the national system, i.e. those that do not require radical upheaval or additional human resources, which they do not want to commit. MSF can be a catalyst in this public health debate, providing that it can provide answers to questions that remain unresolved by using the results of the programme in Bihar, which had already treated over 6,500 children between March 2009 and February 2011.

But the question of the treatment itself is still up for debate and continues to be divisive, even within Right to Food. Progress on this front may well come as a result of an alliance of very different stakeholders. In early 2011, the health authorities and Right to Food members in Madhya Pradesh held talks with the international experts behind the RUTF concept on the possibility of creating a local Indian formula. This alliance has made contact with various local institutions, national food companies and India's food and agriculture cooperatives, one of which, a cooperative with 2.9 million members who are all small-scale producers, boasts the unequivocal slogan: "The Taste of India".

Translated from French by Philippa Bowe-Smith

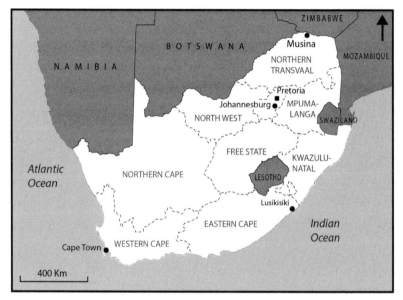

South Africa

SOUTH AFRICA

MSF, AN AFRICAN NGO?

Michaël Neuman

On the eve of the new millennium, Médecins Sans Frontières launched programmes providing access to antiretroviral (ARV) treatment for HIV-infected people. Although national and international initiatives for promoting access to treatment were evolving rapidly at the time, there were still major barriers in the poorest countries, particularly in Africa. The priority was prevention, mainly because of the high price of medicines (between 10,000 and 15,000 dollars per treatment and per year for triple therapies in 2000), but also because existing medical infrastructures and education levels were considered not to be of the necessary standard.[1] Some argued that Africans wouldn't be able to take medication at the right time because "...many people in Africa have never seen a clock or a watch in their entire lives".[2] However, MSF saw South Africa and its sound medical infrastructure as the appropriate setting in which to prove that treating the sick was possible. More than five million people in the country were infected with HIV and had no access to treatment other than that provided at a handful of private facilities.

In 1999, Dr Eric Goemaere, former executive director of the Belgian section of MSF, arrived in South Africa to investigate the opportunity of opening a project for preventing mother-to-child transmission of the HIV virus (PMTCT). After first being stonewalled by the national authorities, he met Zackie Achmat, one of the founders of the Treatment Action Campaign (TAC), a movement formed the previous year by a small group of activists from the anti-apartheid movement to advocate for access to treatment for people with AIDS. Zackie Achmat pointed Eric Goemaere in the direction of Khayelitsha, a township on the outskirts of Cape Town, where the Western Cape Province medical authorities had set up a pilot PMTCT project without the knowledge of the South African Ministry of Health. Khayelitsha had more than 500,000 inhabitants and the HIV prevalence rate among pregnant women was 15%, twice that of the province as a whole.[3] MSF was also interested in the Western Cape because of its unique political context. The province was in the hands of the opposition and MSF felt that this might afford them some room for manoeuvre. Indeed, the new provincial authorities saw in the lack of access to the new treatment options a means of shoring up their criticisms of the ANC (African National Congress).

In February 2000, MSF and TAC joined forces to set up a programme to treat opportunistic diseases, a programme linked to an AIDS education and information project, which involved the patients themselves. In order to pressure the South African authorities into extending the provision of HIV/AIDS care, MSF and TAC considered it crucial for the programme to be owned by poor and black patients, judged by both organisations to be the legitimate voice of contestation in the domain. In this respect, and inspired by contacts with organisations such as Act Up, the movement was continuing in the wake of the European and American activists of the 1980s who had wanted to "challenge the asymmetric relationship between doctor and patient, occupying the domain of the former to make the latter actors in their own treatment".[4] The movement escalated, resonating with a South African society whose capacity for mobilisation and politicisation was a legacy of the anti-apartheid struggle.

When the Cause Justifies the Alliance

In 2001, the outcome of the Pretoria Trial put an end to the South African government using the high cost of medicines as a reason for the lack of access to treatment: the pharmaceutical companies that had accused it of not complying with international rules on the protection of intellectual property dropped their lawsuit, opening the way for the use of generic medicines.

From then on it became clear that the absence of treatment in public healthcare facilities was in fact due to opposition on the part of the South African authorities themselves. President Thabo Mbeki and his health minister Dr Manto Tshabalala-Msimang, increasingly open in their support for arguments refuting the link between AIDS and HIV, had begun promoting "natural" remedies.

This policy of "denialism"[5] found favour among some members of South Africa's ruling classes, seduced by the pipe dream of developing their own drug and a racial interpretation of AIDS, seeing it as a means for whites to perpetuate their domination.[6] These were the beliefs that TAC was fighting, a battle to which MSF contributed its medical legitimacy drawn from the fast-developing project in Khayelitsha, along with its international visibility and financial support. The project introduced antiretrovirals (ARVs) in May 2001 and so, for the first time in South Africa, ARVs were accessible to AIDS patients in public healthcare facilities.

Operating as an alliance was essential to the success of the fight and crucial for increasing the number of patients receiving treatment, not only for Fareed Abdullah, provincial director of the AIDS programmes in Cape Province, but also for MSF and TAC. The University of Cape Town's School of Public Health provided the necessary scientific endorsement and became co-owner of the data produced by the project. At the time, Western Cape was the only province controlled by the political opposition to the ruling ANC, an opposition mainly constituted of white liberals from the anti-apartheid movement. There was, therefore, a real risk of the project being hijacked for political ends. Yet neither MSF nor TAC was opposed to the ANC; Fareed Abdullah was a former ANC executive and in this capacity launched the pilot project when the province was still under ANC control. So MSF played the multipartite card, allowing different political representatives to claim part of the credit. Nelson Mandela himself was of great help as, not only did he support TAC's demands, but in 2002, while the controversy was at its height, he travelled to Khayelitsha where he visited the MSF project, openly defying the government's policy. In 2003, MSF and the Nelson Mandela Foundation opened a joint HIV project in the rural ANC-controlled town of Lusikisiki in Eastern Cape Province.

TAC and, in particular, Zackie Achmat, using their long-standing allegiance to the ANC as an argument for opposing the government, succeeded in creating a broad social movement in support of their combat and organised numerous demonstrations, gatherings and civil disobedience campaigns—including the occupation of public buildings. Drawing on the highly progressive South African Constitution of 1996, the organisation won a number of battles, including setting up a national PMTCT programme (2001 to 2002) and a national AIDS response programme (2004). Given that the Constitution provided for a legally enforceable right to healthcare, the activists were able to use the courts as a political arena. Publically at least, MSF kept its distance from most of these battles, an attitude which its partners found difficult to understand. But TAC's own agenda, as well as its close relations with highly politicised organisations such as the powerful trade union federation close to the ANC, COSATU, was sufficient justification for this in the eyes of the organisation. As it was, MSF was already dealing with numerous accusations of political interference. In 2002, for example, a government spokesperson described the organisation's importing of generic antiretrovirals from Brazil as "a form of bacteriological warfare".[7] It was also accused of using the funding of TAC's activities in Khayelitsha and Lusikisiki as a means of manipulating the movement.[8]

For MSF, a broad range of alliances—a classic tactic of the anti-apartheid struggle—was a condition for success. At a time when the country had just rid itself of white power, MSF could hardly draw legitimacy from its identity as an organisation from the "North". Thus, the alliances built by MSF were a means of gaining the space it needed to develop its activity and advocate for access to treatment. These alliances also became a political shield, essential for warding off attempts by the South African government to destabilise the Khayelitsha programme. Indeed, it was a patient support group that wrote to Thabo Mbeki in response to the attacks by his spokesperson,[9] publishing its letter in the press.

When the Alliance Justifies the Cause

The benefits that MSF gained from its collaboration and from the relations it developed with South African civil society encouraged it to push the experience further and, in 2007, it was decided an office would be opened in Johannesburg. This move was part of a plan by MSF Belgium to internationalise MSF, as the movement's many centres were mostly situated in the "North" (Europe, United States and Canada). Locally, the aim was to involve South African society and, more broadly, that of the southern African sub-region, in MSF's activities and to "continue to draw from the reservoir of ideas generated by a society mobilised to respond to public health issues". South Africa thus became a laboratory for the organisation which went on to test "just how activist it should be".[10] Brussels decided to appoint a South African woman, a former anti-apartheid activist with close ties to TAC and COSATU and highly committed to social and political causes, to head its new office. Although reporting to Brussels, the office in Johannesburg was firmly anchored in the civil society from whence it came. But it had no control over MSF's operations in South Africa, which were still directed by MSF Belgium's head office.

Until this point, MSF's focus in South Africa was exclusively on the response to AIDS, but this was to change considerably with the emergence of the issue of Zimbabwean migrants, which fuelled one of the organisation's recurrent controversies: how much activism can the organisation justify in the name of its medical and humanitarian expertise? In 2006, fleeing economic hardship, repression and political violence, 1.5 to three million Zimbabweans began arriving in South Africa. Tens of thousands of them were turned back at the border whilst others settled down to a precarious existence in the country. In December 2007, MSF opened projects on the Zimbabwean border and in Johannesburg, where it provided medical consultations to between 2,000 and 3,000 Zimbabweans who had found refuge in a Methodist church and in abandoned buildings in the surrounding area.

The discussions between MSF and its partners were quickly to move beyond the strict confines of access to healthcare. This had been a legal entitlement for foreigners since 2007, although it was still constrained by fear of arrest, staff shortages and the language barrier—sometimes used as a pretext for refusing them access to medical facilities. Between 2008 and 2010, within the framework of a partnership with a number of lawyers' organisations (notably Lawyers for Human Rights and AIDS Law Project) and the church's Methodist priest, MSF became actively involved in the issue of migrants' rights, with the aim of making sure their voices were heard. A project was launched with "the express purpose of bringing about political change".[11] The partners shared the roles between them: MSF, the constitution of medical expertise; and the lawyers the capacity to run campaigns using the information supplied to them. The network, established during previous combats—including the AIDS response—was fully mobilised. Once again, the South African constitution provided the ammunition necessary for taking political contestation before the courts.

On several occasions between 2008 and 2010, MSF worked alongside its allies to promote the rights of migrants. In 2009, in response to migrants gathered around the church, some of whom were queuing up for a medical consultation, the project coordinator agreed to sign a written testimony describing the medical conditions of people under arrest to enable human rights organisations to file a complaint against the city and the police. By drawing on the South African Constitution, the organisations succeeded in putting a stop to arrests for vagrancy. This action was at its height during the xenophobic violence of May 2008 when the foreigners living in displacement camps were threatened with expulsion. MSF was denied access to the camps where its mobile teams had been providing daily consultations. The organisation issued a press release denouncing the apathy of the UNHCR and the fact that its position was founded on international conventions,[12] whereas MSF and its allies based themselves on the South African Constitution. On each of these occasions, controversy arose within the mission, as well as between the mission, the South African office and headquarters in Brussels, on the limits to the role and responsibilities of MSF.

MSF's potential support for a "Declaration concerning the resolution of the refugees crisis", initiated by the Aids Law Project, Lawyers for Human Rights and the Legal Resources Centre, and to which a very large and very diverse group of organisations adhered, was the subject of heated debate in December 2009. Whereas the South African office wanted MSF to support the declaration, which called for respect of the rights of Zimbabweans living in Zimbabwe and condemnation of the actions of President Mugabe, at headquarters in Brussels the organisation was opposed, arguing that this would be "crossing the line".[13] Both the mission and Brussels criticised the charges laid against the Zimbabwean regime and the disparate nature of the signatures, and argued that open opposition to the government in Harare would jeopardise MSF's activities in Zimbabwe. For its part, the office in Johannesburg explained that leaving the coalition could undermine MSF's position in South Africa by distancing it from the progressist battles being fought by its traditional allies. Indeed, for these allies, defending the rights of migrants or the right to medical treatment was consistent with their ambition to make their presence felt at all social and political levels in South Africa. MSF was not ready to take this step, did not support the declaration, but made one of its own. It considered that the limits to the organisation's legitimate scope of intervention had been reached.

Translated from French by Mandy Duret

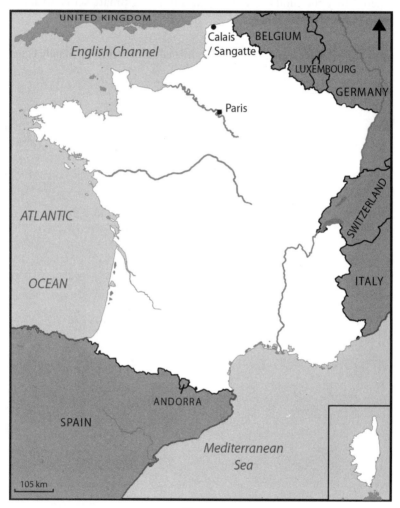

France

FRANCE

MANAGING THE "UNDESIRABLES"

Michaël Neuman

In France, the emergence of a "new poverty"[1] led Médecins Sans Frontières to turn its attention to the country's medical and political arenas in 1987. Developing activities such as free healthcare, dentistry and prevention of lead poisoning, MSF, "in its capacity as French doctors and as a medical organisation operating in France",[2] sought to alert the authorities to the shortcomings in access to healthcare for the most vulnerable of French citizens and foreign nationals. The organisation, refusing to become a substitute for the state, chose to restrict its healthcare centres to a number sufficient to enable it to play the role of alerting the authorities. Various different stands were taken by MSF over time: calling for state healthcare coverage to be extended to all categories of people in 1991, denouncing the refusal to hospitalise people without state healthcare coverage in 1993, and opposing the creation of respite beds[3] in 1994, which was seen as a parallel healthcare system for the poor, whereas MSF was seeking to reintegrate them into the mainstream healthcare system.

A new project was launched in 1996 "to offer advice on social services and legal support to foreign nationals living in France". This initiative endorsed MSF's ambition to "break with the charity role" that had characterised it from its inception, even if it meant venturing into "non medical and uncharted" territory.[4] It became actively involved—

through legislative reform—in providing legal support to people deprived of access to healthcare, by contributing to drawing up the law on the Couverture Maladie Universelle (universal healthcare coverage, or CMU), and taking legal action to ensure application of people's entitlement to medical aid, which led to proceedings against the Nord and the Bouches-du-Rhône local councils.

The adoption of the CMU law in July 1999[5] was the culmination of a programme driven by people determined to challenge public policy. Nearly four million people benefit from the CMU, which resolves the majority of problems in access to healthcare. But no sooner had the public health issue lost its urgency, than surfaced the question of the mission's new direction. In 2001, it was noted that, "access to rights will remain an important part of MSF's programmes in France, but [that] this issue alone can no longer justify maintaining existing programmes or opening new centres".[6] MSF launched new initiatives, particularly in the area of accommodation, and continued to monitor application of Aide Médicale d'État (state medical aid, or AME)[7] and the repercussions of its successive reforms. In 2003, Mission France underwent a radical overhaul, justified in part by the will to reduce the cost of projects. This development coincided with MSF scaling down its objectives to run what were known as "access to healthcare and exclusion" programmes and refocusing on operational policies targeting "direct victims of violence", considered a priority in the allocation of resources.

Thus the projects were gradually closed down, since there was no "health emergency"[8] that would have justified MSF setting up medical activities. The major public health issues of the mid-1980s had mostly been resolved. The CMU and the AME, in spite of some malfunctions and the adoption of restrictive measures, played the role they were supposed to; from 1998, some 400 Permanences d'accès aux soins (healthcare access centres, or PASS) were set up in public hospitals throughout France to provide the most disadvantaged with access to healthcare. However, while MSF could have considered putting an end to its mission, the tightening of asylum policies in France and Europe and the consequences for migrants' health justified, on the contrary, new actions. In 2006, the association set up a walk-in clinic for refugees in Sangatte in northern France, and then closed it after a healthcare access centre that it had helped to establish opened at nearby Calais hospital. MSF went on to open a "support and healthcare centre" in Paris in 2007 to provide psychological care to asylum seekers (particularly non-French speakers) suffering from psychological problems. The centre also offers social and legal advice. The organisation undertook a number of evaluations that disclosed the inadequacies in the treatment of psychological trauma, arising as much from the asylum seekers' personal stories as from their battles with red tape.

The avowed political dimension of the project drew on the 1951 Convention relating to the status of refugees and which defines the rights of asylum seekers, particularly in terms of non-refoulement (repatriation). Its advocates saw it as raising the profile of "this humanitarian issue [...] by highlighting the interaction between medical status and access to refuge".[9] MSF's president opposed the project, challenging the existence of an "asylum crisis", questioning the feasibility of the medical objectives and denouncing inconsistencies in operational decisions: accepting today what had seemingly been refused yesterday, i.e., caring for a few at a high cost—one of the reasons behind closing projects in the past.[10] Others challenged MSF's legitimacy in taking a stand on the issue of the right to asylum and, by extension, on the government's immigration policy, exposing major divisions within the organisation on the subject.

The exchanges of views preceding the launch of the project were a presage of the difficulties to come, as they revealed the differences of opinion on MSF's legitimacy in shifting from the humanitarian sector to the social sector. In answer to some of its members' concerns that the organisation was engaging in a political battle too far removed from its field of expertise, those behind the project made every effort not to appear involved in a movement to oppose the government's immigration policy.[11] Limiting confrontation with the authorities, they stepped up the number of medical consultations in order to increase legitimacy and accumulate experience and information. Medico-psychological activities provided an answer to real problems, in this case, functional disorders—even if they only helped a small number of people (900 between March 2007 and December 2010). In addition, MSF's objective to confront the authorities was restricted by the limited scope of the medical field the organisation could draw from. A number of opportunities for challenging the authorities were seized, but without finding a more general framework to work within. The health safety net provided by the authorities rendered the project's position particularly complex, since there is little doubt that from the perspective of the French government there was never any question of leaving undocumented immigrants to die.

As Eric Besson, then minister for immigration, said in the spring of 2009: "Humanitarian action to help foreigners in distress, regardless of their residency status, is perfectly legal".[12] In a letter to NGOs, he specified that the state, "along with local authorities, [was providing] major technical and financial support—over 20 million euros a year—to organisations providing assistance to undocumented immigrants, and their humanitarian role is vital".[13] The government thus applied an increasingly clear distinction between "good" humanitarian organisations, providing assistance and compassionate treatment to "superfluous" people reduced to silence, and "bad" activist and political organisations seeking to "give a voice to the excluded poor".[14] So, humanitarian action was legitimate, as long as it did not lead to any criticism of public policy.[15]

By treating individual suffering[16] and not questioning the political and social origins of such suffering too closely, is MSF not confining itself to the role expected of it by the authorities: in other words, playing into their hands by looking after people rejected by the system? Avoiding the pitfall of shared management with the authorities of those deemed "undesirable" necessarily means making good use of MSF's role as an expert in the conflicts it believes it should legitimately be involved in. However, the extent of the health safety net in France curbs the organisation's potential for criticism, putting it at risk of compassionate treatment of individual suffering. In autumn 2010, parliamentary and governmental offensives against the AME and the right to residency of foreign nationals in ill health did, however, give MSF new reason to take a stand in an area where it feels legitimate. These stances were justified by the role the organisation had played in setting up some of the systems, as well as concerns as to possible consequences of the reforms on people's health.

Translated from French by Philippa Bowe-Smith

PART TWO

HISTORY

SILENCE HEALS...

FROM THE COLD WAR TO THE WAR ON TERROR, MSF SPEAKS OUT: A BRIEF HISTORY

Fabrice Weissman

In a growing number of countries such as Ethiopia, Russia, Zimbabwe and Sri Lanka, national laws and government framework agreements oblige MSF to strict confidentiality. These restrictions are causing some discomfort within the organisation, which claims the right to "speak out and bear witness", and its leaders are being forced to take a new look at an issue that has been under debate since its inception: why get involved in the public debate? Shaped by experiences in the field and the dominant ideological currents, MSF's responses have evolved over the past forty years. Here we'd like to give a brief history of the major positions taken by the organisation during conflicts, within a context marked successively by the Cold War, the collapse of the bipolar world order, and the increase in armed international intervention in the name of human rights.

1970 to 1980: Choosing Neo-conservatism

The Good Samaritans of Disaster

Contrary to the image popularised by the media and MSF itself, the idea that silence was necessary to action was held by a majority of its founding members. The original charter of 1971 stipulated that its members would refrain from "any interference in States' internal affairs" and abstain from "passing judgment or publicly expressing an opinion—either positive or negative—regarding events, forces or leaders who accepted their assistance". When asked during an interview by French newspaper *l'Est Républicain* on 26 December 1971, "Should a doctor who witnesses atrocities remain silent?", MSF co-founder and fire brigade colonel Dr Gérard Pigeon replied in the affirmative: "We have to be perfectly clear: doctors don't go to be witnesses. They don't go to write a novel or a newspaper article; they go to treat. Doctor-patient privilege exists, and should be respected. If doctors keep quiet, they'll be allowed in; otherwise they'll be kept out like everyone else".

From 1971 to 1976, the fledgling organisation promoted a depoliticised image showcasing the courage of its members and the technical efficacy of its medical care. It wasn't until 1977 that an MSF representative first violated the statutory confidentiality commitment. On returning from the Cambodian refugee camps along the Thai border, Claude Malhuret condemned, on France's leading television station,[1] the "revolutionary crimes" of the Khmer Rouge who, he said, were "exterminating entire segments of the population in the name of some revamped communist ideology". The MSF archives reveal nothing of the discussions that were prompted by this speaking out, which sparked controversy and led to the organisation receiving several letters accusing its leaders of being propagandists on the payroll of the CIA. In any event, in 1977–78, the commitment to confidentiality was officially challenged by MSF directors. In 1978, the president announced in his annual report that staff would be "reporting human rights violations and unacceptable events they witnessed to the bureau. (...) The bureau will then make an executive decision on whether to inform the public, in cases where MSF was the sole witness".

While the majority at MSF were in favour of "the right to speak out", the leadership team was torn about the place it should have. Bernard Kouchner and some of the other founders viewed it as the primary function of Médecins Sans Frontières, which needed to guard against becoming "bureaucrats of misery and technocrats of charity".[2] Action was the responsibility of the (democratic) governments, and all MSF could do was to galvanise them by creating a stir in the media. Malhuret, on the other hand, wanted to anchor speaking out in the independent and effective practice of humanitarian medicine, which meant professionalising the organisation. Finding himself in the minority, Bernard Kouchner left MSF in 1979.

The Cambodian March for Survival

The new leadership team immediately put the "right to speak out" into action in Cambodia in 1979 to 1980. Convinced that the country was in the grip of a famine and that the pro-Vietnamese regime was diverting humanitarian aid, MSF demanded an internationally-monitored, large-scale distribution of aid based on cross-border access from Thailand. To that end, on 20 December 1979 MSF leaders called for a "March for Survival" for Cambodia. On 6 February 1980, about a hundred demonstrators—including Rony Brauman and Claude Malhuret for MSF, Bernard-Henry Lévy for Action Internationale Contre la Faim (AICF), and Joan Baez for the International Rescue Committee (IRC)—showed up at the Cambodian/Thai border at the head of a food convoy. Not surprisingly, they were turned away. More numerous than the demonstrators, journalists gave plenty of coverage to the event, which was criticised by the pro-Vietnamese government and its allies as an imperialist, reactionary demonstration. Dissent also grew within MSF, where some accused the leadership of being manipulated by the United States for propaganda purposes—in particular, by associating with the IRC, which many saw as a front for the CIA.

To those who maintained that MSF should "do humanitarianism, not politics", Malhuret replied, "This is politics in the true sense of the word. People are dying of hunger in Cambodia, and we can't intervene. If you had known about Auschwitz, would you have buried your head in the sand?"[3] This reference to the ICRC's controversial role during World War II was, at the time, a standard feature in the arguments put forward by Malhuret and Brauman, who saw communist totalitarianism as the source of contemporary genocidal processes. In their view, *détente* was just a smokescreen for a vast Soviet offensive in the third world. By the late-1970s, former Indochina was entirely in the hands of Soviet and Chinese allies, Soviet influence extended into Africa

(Angola, Ethiopia, Mozambique, etc.), there were several revolutionary movements in Latin America (Nicaragua, El Salvador and Guatemala), and the Red Army had invaded Afghanistan. In its work with
refugee camp populations—which grew from three million to eleven
million between the late-1970s and early-1980s—MSF found that
90% of them were fleeing from communist regimes.

In terms of its stated operational objectives—ensuring independent
distribution of relief—the Cambodian March for Survival was a failure. However, as the organisation would learn several years later, there
wasn't actually a famine—not because the government distributed the
aid that reached them, but because there was no widespread food
shortage. Contrary to popular opinion, the malnourished state of the
refugees arriving in Thailand which triggered the alert was not representative of the situation inside Cambodia.[4] The march did, however,
put the organisation back in the headlines through a political action
with at least three messages: by demanding independent distribution of
relief supplies, MSF was asserting that, without a minimum amount of
autonomy, aid is condemned to serve the interests of political power at
the population's expense. By addressing itself to public opinion, and
through it to the States themselves, it underscored the fact that such
autonomy can only be won after a power struggle in which the authorities' international image is at stake. By publicising the pro-Vietnamese
government's refusal of independent aid, it showed that autonomy was
non-existent in countries with totalitarian regimes, where aid was destined to be turned into an instrument of oppression. Nine years after
MSF's creation on a foundation of silence and neutrality, its leaders
made speaking out an important part of humanitarian action, supporting and extending aid policies.

The 1980s: The War Against Communism

The condemnation of Red Army crimes in Afghanistan was emblematic of how speaking out can be an extension of medical action. Working with the Afghan resistance since 1981, MSF had to cope with
logistical and security constraints due not only to the clandestine
nature of its mission, but also to the tribal, political and military strategies of the Afghan faction heads. "Relations with the Mujahedin gave
us infinitely more trouble than the Red Army",[5] commented Juliette
Fournot, the mission's main organiser. Yet MSF did not openly criticise

the obstacles imposed by the Afghan resistance; it condemned the Soviet occupation forces for massive bombing, dropping antipersonnel mines, and setting fire to villages and crops. "We were helping more people by denouncing what was happening over there than by offering assistance to the few Afghans we were able to get to. By alerting the public, we were making politicians face up to their responsibility, and forcing them to intervene to stop the massacre",[6] explained Malhuret, years later.

To the MSF leadership, in the context of the Cold War, "making politicians face up to their responsibility" meant calling upon the liberal democracies to redouble their efforts in the fight against communism.[7] To this end, Malhuret made several trips to the United States between 1983 and 1985, at the invitation of neo-conservative intellectuals and Republican Senator Gordon J. Humphrey. Humphrey was one of the promoters of Operation Cyclone, the CIA programme that equipped and funded the Afghan resistance from 1979 to 1989. Media coverage of MSF's Afghanistan activities and accounts of its experiences then became part of the moral rearmament effort launched in the mid-1970s by neo-conservative intellectuals and the US administration. Taking advantage of the new political infatuation with human rights in an America seeking moral purification (the religious revival, the public's discomfort with the atrocities committed in Vietnam, and the Watergate scandal), they used the human rights movement in the ideological war against communism, supporting Soviet dissidents, Polish trade union Solidarity, the signatories of the Charter 77 in Czechoslovakia, etc.[8] MSF received several rounds of funding from the National Endowment for Democracy (NED), a foundation designed to export American "soft power" through civil society organisations.

The NED got what they paid for. In 1984, MSF created the Liberté Sans Frontières (LSF) Foundation, a think-tank on development and human rights issues. The LSF scientific committee was made up of liberal-right Atlanticist thinkers, most of them from the editorial board of Raymond Aron's journal, *Commentaire*. In 1985, LSF held a symposium entitled "Third Worldism in Question", during which it lambasted what it considered the ready-made ideology of the aid world: Third Worldism that sought to justify the NGOs' blindly lining up behind the China- or Soviet-allied governments of newly independent states in the name of anti-imperialism. "LSF discourse is deeply imbued with the ideologies it claims to be emancipated from; it is not located outside [any framework] but anchored in a Reaganist, pro-American thinking", commented Alain Gresh in May 1985, in a special issue of *Le Monde Diplomatique*.

"Aid is Used to Oppress, Not to Save"

At the same time as it was condemning the crimes of totalitarianism, during the 1980s MSF spoke out in an attempt to extract itself from situations where it believed humanitarian aid was "having a perverse effect" to the point of becoming "complicit in criminal policies".[9] In 1984–85, there was a famine followed by a large relief operation in Ethiopia financed by the western nations and private donors, mobilised by an unprecedented media campaign which culminated in the Live Aid concert, organised by Bob Geldof. In the first half of 1985, MSF— which was running nutrition and hospital programmes in several camps sheltering tens of thousands of people fleeing the famine—came to realise that the food distribution centres were traps. The government was using the food aid as blackmail, giving it only to families that agreed to participate in a relocation programme aimed mainly at depopulating rebel areas by moving people from the north to the south. Those who refused to go were taken at gunpoint.

According to MSF estimates, at least 100,000 people died while being transferred or during the first three months of resettlement. It launched a public opinion campaign in September 1985, calling upon donors and humanitarian organisations—unsuccessfully—to form a united front in demanding a moratorium on the deportations, which would kill more people than the famine itself. A month later, MSF was expelled from Ethiopia.

While this denunciation ultimately merged with MSF's condemnation of totalitarianism's disasters, it came out of a very different process than the public stands on Afghanistan. The intent was not to prolong emergency relief, but to challenge its use in the service of murderous policies. MSF used public opinion to pressure the UN, NGOs, and western nations; the aim was to transform their aid practices, to prevent them from stepping over "that blurry, but very real, line beyond which assistance for victims imperceptibly turns into support for their tormentors".[10]

In the end, by condemning communist totalitarianism as the root of the greatest human disasters and for using humanitarian action against its beneficiaries, MSF made common cause with the west during the Cold War. It saw its action as a part of the fight for human rights and democracy: "Though imperfect, the [liberal political systems] are the only ones in history that have allowed significant advances in freedoms and social justice".[11] In the same vein, the association applied for the Council of Europe Human Rights Prize in 1988. Believing that the award would constitute "a moral recognition giving more weight to [its] interventions in the Third World",[12] it pointed out that, "since its beginnings, MSF has acted to promote and defend human rights": by its action, it responds to the "right of populations to have access to medical care", and by its presence, it acts as "a decisive deterrent in preventing human rights abuses". Lastly, it reserved the "right to speak out publicly on atrocities about which its teams have knowledge, when they are alone in a place where outside observers cannot investigate".[13] Presented every three years, the prize was awarded to Lech Walesa in 1989; MSF won it in 1992.

The 1990s: The Gamble of Liberal Internationalism

The Hope for a "New World Order Based on Human Rights"

With the end of the Cold War, speaking out publicly and defending human rights began to gain some legitimacy within the other four sections of MSF. Created during the 1980s in Belgium, Holland, Spain and Switzerland, they had until then resolutely opposed the French practice of bearing witness, which they accused of politicising MSF in violation of its statutes. After bitter debate, in 1992 all of the sections decided to remove the provisions in the charter committing MSF to confidentiality and prohibiting it from any involvement in a country's internal affairs. Because of the complexity in retracing how speaking out evolved from the 1990s on—characterised by evolving, contradictory messages, heavily influenced by experiences in the field and fiercely debated within the movement—we will give a selective reading, taken primarily from French section experiences.

During the 1990s, there were fewer and fewer refugee camps, and humanitarian aid began to be deployed inside conflict zones. Clandestine missions conducted under guerrilla protection gave way to larger-scale projects requiring agreement from several belligerents. The latter were especially numerous in countries like Somalia and Liberia or, like the governments of Iraq, Myanmar and Sudan, were fundamentally opposed to intervention by western NGOs. Though it had never before been so present in the midst of war, in 1992 MSF considered that, "the main problem today is that of access to victims; the authorities or factions oppose humanitarian action, an inconvenient witness to their atrocities, and insecurity makes intervention increasingly dangerous".[14]

Faced with these difficulties, MSF had to reckon with the resources and constraints inherent to a new type of internationalisation of conflicts. In the five years following the 1991 Gulf War—pitched by the US administration as the first act of a "new world order"—the UN Security Council launched twenty-four peacekeeping missions, as many as there had been in the whole of its first forty-five years of existence. Establishing a link between threats to peace and violations of international humanitarian law, the UN authorised the use of force to safeguard aid operations, particularly in Iraqi Kurdistan, Somalia, and Bosnia. While humanitarian doctors had traditionally followed armies onto the battlefield, "now it is the armies themselves that escort humanitarian organisations to the frontline",[15] observed a perplexed MSF in 1993.

Yet, its directors welcomed the growing involvement of the UN and western nations in the conflicts. With Soviet totalitarianism defeated, the democratic states and the UN would, more than ever, have, "an essential role to play [...] in guaranteeing genuine access to victims and an end to human rights violations".[16] Therefore, MSF increasingly challenged western governments and the UN, criticising in particular military interventions that claimed the protection of humanitarian actors as their mandate. Such interventions did not always improve access to victims. But more than that, they served the western powers as an alibi for avoiding what was, according to MSF, their primary responsibility—combating massive human rights violations, including by military means.

Denunciation of the Humanitarian Alibi

MSF's first critique of the "humanitarian alibi" was in response to the international intervention in Iraq. Taking advantage of the weakened Iraqi regime in the wake of the first Gulf War, Kurds and Shiites rose up in March 1991, only to be crushed by the Republican Guard, which pushed more than a million Kurds into exodus. The displaced piled up at the Iranian and Turkish borders, causing concern in Ankara, which feared a massive influx of Kurds in the provinces where its army was already fighting an insurrection. On 5 April 1991, the Security Council condemned the repression of the Iraqi civilian population as a threat to international peace and security, and demanded that Iraq allow immediate access by international humanitarian organisations to all those in need of assistance. France and the US used their armed forces in a massive, technically successful relief and repatriation operation (Operation Provide Comfort); some sixty NGOs participated, one of them MSF. Nevertheless, the organisation criticised the cynicism with which the western nations—after having encouraged them to rebel—left the Kurds and the Shiites to be massacred. In MSF's view, Operation Provide Comfort served to "disguise the partial failure of a Gulf War unable to put an end to Saddam Hussein's rule".[17]

Implicit in the case of Kurdistan, condemnation of state humanitarianism as an alternative to war against criminal regimes was at the heart of MSF's public opinion campaign during the Bosnian War (1992 to 1995). In addition to killing between 20,000 and 60,000 people,[18] that conflict displaced about two million, roughly half of the population. Prompted by terrorist tactics such as mass killing, torching of villages, executions, rape, and internment, forced displacement was not an indirect consequence of the war, but one of its main objectives. Croatian, Muslim and Serbian nationalists (the last enjoying military superiority, thanks to Yugoslav army support) all nursed more or less radical ambitions for ethnic homogeneity in the territories they claimed.

The utility of MSF medical intervention in the central European country—with its modern healthcare system and qualified medical personnel—was marginal. The organisation focused primarily on helping the displaced and providing medical supplies to Muslim enclaves surrounded by Bosnian Serb forces. "Aside from material assistance, we saw our presence in those besieged towns as a symbolic act: the need to be witnesses", reflected Pierre Salignon, a member of MSF-France's mission in Bosnia.[19]

Witness to the blockade of enclaves packed with thousands of displaced persons and exposed to sniper fire and Serb artillery, and aware of the civilian internment camps and the terrorist methods being used by militias to drive out populations, MSF had no intention of remaining neutral between the besiegers and the besieged, the deported and those organising the deportations. Beginning in April 1992, and then during the June visit to Sarajevo by French president François Mitterrand—who explained that French and UN involvement would be limited to protecting humanitarian aid—MSF heads stepped up their statements to the press. They criticised the "passivity of the international community" and, more particularly, of European countries, in the face of the "ethnic cleansing" in Bosnia. For MSF, ethnic homogenisation of certain areas by Serb militias signalled the resurgence of genocidal totalitarianism in the heart of Europe. This is why MSF considered humanitarian action by NGOs to be derisory, if not complicit, given its role of accompanying—even helping—a criminal policy.[20] In 1992, the French section suggested that the entire movement halt all its operations in Bosnia. As Rony Brauman declared on French radio station RTL in April 1992, "It's the hills of Sarajevo that should be bombed. We should declare war on the Serb nationalists".[21]

In addition to the spectre of genocide, MSF's call to arms was anchored in international humanitarian law. In November 1992, the teams conducted a survey—the first of its kind—among sixty or so Bosnian refugees in France. Seeking to retrace the history of their flight and give a legal definition to the violence they survived, the report on the "process of ethnic cleansing in the Kazarac region" concluded that "the atrocities committed by the Serbs of Bosnia-Herzegovina were not just human rights violations or war crimes, but a crime against humanity, according to the definition of the Nuremberg Tribunal". The report was distributed to the press and to numerous institutions, such as the US Congress and the United Nations Special Rapporteur for Yugoslavia. The call to arms took the form of an appeal for an "international policing operation (...); governments have the duty to use all necessary means to halt serious violations of humanitarian law".[22]

By demanding that western governments make war against oppressive regimes, rather than protect relief operations, MSF entered the public debate alongside neo-conservatives and liberal internationalists. Since the fall of the Berlin Wall, the latter insisted that liberal democracies had a responsibility, and an interest, in using their military power to defend human rights beyond their borders. Surprisingly, MSF's pro-Bosnian involvement did not seem to provoke direct reprisals by the Serb militias, with whom it had to negotiate its presence in the former Yugoslavia. The neo-conservative rhetoric it helped amplify, however, was sharply criticised by Bosnia-Herzegovina specialists as a factor in the radicalisation of the conflict. This call to arms, which painted Serb nationalism as a contemporary form of Nazism, encouraged the military escalation and use of the victim strategy by Croatian nationalists and Muslims suspected of deliberately exposing their civilian populations in order to get armed support from the west.[23]

Somalia, Rwanda: "People were Killed Under the Banner of Humanitarianism"

MSF interventionism was, however, shaken in Somalia, where the association realised that the international military remedy could turn out to be worse than the disease. The primary mandate of the American and UN troops landing in Mogadishu in 1992–93 was to safeguard humanitarian relief operations in a context of famine and widespread insecurity. The arrival of foreign forces was met with ambivalence by MSF. The Belgian section was officially in favour, seeing it as a way "to gain access to rural areas, to guarantee [humanitarian organisations] more effective protection" as well as "an end to the vicious cycle of paying militias". With the collapse of the Somali government and the privatisation of violence, MSF was, in effect, forced to hire the services of armed guards made available by warlords, whom it was thus directly funding, prompting criticism from journalists and staff. The French and Dutch sections, on the other hand, were more sceptical of the international troops' highly publicised arrival, believing that the strategy of dialogue and negotiation hitherto used by the United Nations Special Representative was more likely to create conditions conducive to expanding relief activities.

In the early months of 1993, the international deployment allowed more food aid distributions in the interior of the country, which helped to contain the already-declining famine. But the international forces quickly became party to the conflict, committing countless atrocities, including the bombing of hospitals and local relief organisations, the torture and killing of non-combatants, and civilian massacres. Associated in people's minds with the international forces, humanitarian organisations were being targeted by the factions against whom the UN and US had declared war. The French section withdrew from the country in 1993, condemning the "military-humanitarian confusion" that had put them in danger and the perversion of humanitarian logic. "In Somalia, people were killed for the first time under the banner of humanitarianism".[24] The experience convinced MSF that international

armed protection was a trap, and that once a government has collapsed, the only political objective of military intervention is an international protectorate—with its colonialist overtones and impossible
political and financial costs.[25]

After the experience in Somalia, MSF sketched out its first public critique of international military interventionism. It underscored its limits, its potential for degenerating into brutal war, and the perverse
effects on relief workers, who were seen as no different than the soldiers charged with protecting them. These reservations would be swept
aside, however, by the extraordinarily grave crisis that devastated central Africa's Great Lakes region from 1994 to 1997.

Calls to Arms

Between April and July 1994, Rwanda's Tutsi population was systematically hunted down and exterminated. Working in several Rwandan
towns, MSF gradually became aware of the genocidal nature of the
massacres. Though genocide was expressly denied by United Nations
Security Council members—who had, for various reasons, decided not
to intervene—MSF, for the first time in its history, launched an explicit
appeal for international armed intervention against a regime conducting "the planned, methodical extermination of a community".[26] In the
latter half of 1994, MSF protested the reconstitution of the genocidal
administration in Rwandan refugee camps with close to two million
people in Zaire and Tanzania. While the UN secretary general was not
able to assemble the forces needed to neutralise the genocidal network,
MSF called upon the UN and western powers to demilitarise the
camps, provide policing, and arrest the organisers behind the genocide.
The failure of these efforts convinced the organisation to leave the
camps between 1994 and 1995, in order not to be "accomplices of the
genocide's perpetrators",[27] against whom it had called for war.

A year later, the camps in Zaire were attacked one after the other by
the new Rwandan regime's army and its Congolese allies. After returning to the region in November 1996, MSF once again called for armed
international intervention, "to protect the refugees and guarantee
access to aid". But, arguing that large numbers of refugees had
returned to Rwanda, the western nations declared the crisis over and
the intervention never happened. Several hundred thousand Rwandans
refused to return to their country, however. They were hunted down

mercilessly by the Rwandan army and its Congolese allies, who used humanitarian organisations as bait to attract those who fled—not to deport them, as in Ethiopia, but to physically eradicate them. Throughout 1997, MSF publicly condemned the massacres and human rights violations that its teams had knowledge of, without any real success in prompting efforts to stop the killers.

In 1997, recalling that MSF had done everything it could to try to "humanise the inhuman", the president of MSF-France acknowledged the limits of the organisation's actions and public statements in the face of extreme violence: "We tried to do the least possible harm".[28] From the mid-1990s, the post-Cold War euphoria fuelling hope for a "new world order based on human rights"[29] gave way to somewhat bitter caution. As Philippe Biberson declared at the 1996 General Assembly, "One must beware of the megalomaniacal vision which aims to wage a universal struggle for justice and democracy and of the UN's vision of well-being shared by all". MSF began to refocus its public stance on assistance policies and distance itself from liberal interventionism, entrusting the UN—backed by the western democracies—with the responsibility for ensuring respect for human rights on a global scale.

1999 and Beyond: Navigating Between Imperialism and Despotism

"Blurring of Lines"

As MSF was questioning the significance of its appeals to the UN and western nations, the number of international military interventions was growing. In March 1999, NATO launched a campaign of air strikes against the Federal Republic of Yugoslavia, forcing the Serb army terrorising the Albanian-speaking population of Kosovo to withdraw. Five months later, Australian troops landed in East Timor under the UN flag, putting an end to atrocities by pro-Indonesian militias opposed to independence for the former Portuguese colony. In May 2000, a contingent of British paratroopers joined UN troops deployed in Sierra Leone, helping to bring a fragile calm to the country devastated by ten years of civil war. A year later, the September 11 2001 attacks against the United States were followed by the invasions of Afghanistan in 2001, and Iraq in 2003. At the same time, UN peacekeeping operations were stepped up, as their mandate now included protecting civilian populations inter alia and not just humanitarian relief operations.[30] With 140,000 soldiers and police deployed in sixteen countries, by 2006, UN forces became the second largest army operating on foreign soil, after that of the United States.

This resurgence in interventionism was rationalised by security concerns (protecting democracy from global threats such as pandemics, migration, organised crime, terrorism, etc.) and humanitarian considerations (combating mass human rights violations and freeing populations from want and oppression). As British Prime Minister Tony Blair declared in April 1999, "we [Europe and the US] cannot turn our backs on conflicts and the violation of human rights within other countries if we want still to be secure". The new secretary general of the UN, Kofi Annan, justified sending Australian troops to East Timor in terms of the member States' responsibility to collectively assert the primacy of human rights over national sovereignty. Urging the Security Council to adopt a doctrine of intervention—"the responsibility to protect"—that would authorise the use of force in response "to a Rwanda, to a Srebrenica—to gross and systematic violations of human rights",[31] he characterised as "historic" the 1 July 2002 creation of the International Criminal Court, the first permanent court charged with trying the perpetrators of war crimes against humanity and genocide.[32]

Asserting that the UN and western powers shared the same aims as the humanitarian organisations, institutional donors suggested that the latter abandon their neutrality and join the political and military coalitions being steered from New York and Washington. With the exception of Iraq, where European and American NGOs disagreed on the appropriateness of using force, many allied themselves with the international troops and participated in stabilisation policies (in Kosovo, Sierra Leone, Afghanistan, the DRC, etc.). Many felt that in this way they were contributing to "the only truly humanitarian goal: hastening the end of a war" and "replacing a murderous regime by a civilized government as quickly as possible" (in the words of former humanitarian volunteer and academic Michael Barry, on Afghanistan).[33]

Beginning with the NATO intervention in Kosovo, MSF declared itself neutral in all conflicts where international forces were involved. It vigorously criticised the notion of "humanitarian war" evoked by Tony Blair and NATO, seeing it as a formula that "makes it easier to forget the human cost arising from the use of force and the political repercussions of violating state sovereignty".[34] Using humanitarianism to justify war weakens democratic debate and exposes aid organisations to the risks of military-humanitarian confusion. In the organisation's view, that confusion was being exacerbated by the involvement of foreign armies in civilian relief efforts, and the fact that those armies presented psychological warfare operations as humanitarian assistance. Such practices cast doubt on the independence and impartiality of humanitarian NGOs, no longer seen as outsiders to the conflict by either the population or the belligerents opposed to the presence of international troops. The criticism became even more extreme after the June 2004 murder of five MSF members in Afghanistan.

Wherever international forces were involved, MSF would judge what it considered correct or incorrect uses of humanitarian semantics, condemning the "blurring of lines" at every level—such-and-such a war was not "humanitarian", certain aid was not "humanitarian", certain NGOs were not "humanitarian"—without, however, demonstrating by its operations or public positions the independence it was proclaiming. In Afghanistan and Iraq, for example, it lost interest in the victims of the war on terror. Aside from some isolated statements by the president of MSF-France, it remained silent in the face of the November 2001 massacres of thousands of prisoners of war by Coalition forces and their Afghan allies—massacres that prompted no demand for an international investigation. It said nothing about the US administration's legalisation of torture, nor did it try to provide care for the victims released from Abu-Ghraib prison. It did not protest when allied forces rejected the distinction between combatants and non-combatants, considering it obsolete in the "war on terror"—an argument taken up in particular by the governments of Russia, Colombia, Algeria, Pakistan and Sri Lanka, which accused NGOs that criticised them of having a double standard.

From 1998 to 2003, however, MSF was extremely critical of the lack of interest shown by the UN and its member states in the violence in Chechnya, Liberia, Algeria, and Colombia, where warring factions enjoyed a "license to kill",[35] thus reducing the population's chances of survival and humanitarian organisations' ability to help them. It also denounced the inability of relief operations to save the victims of war and famine in North Korea (1996–98) and in Sudan (1998), due to their subjugation to crisis management strategies dictated by the foreign policies of the biggest institutional donors (United States, European Union and Japan).

"MSF and Protection—Pending or Closed?"[36]

Yet, by publicly exposing war crimes and the misappropriation or obstruction of humanitarian assistance, MSF may in fact have been encouraging the use of international military or legal measures against the perpetrators. This new dimension of speaking out prompted quite different reactions within each section.

Some were pleased; in the view of one MSF lawyer, the threat of legal (and military) action was "sharper teeth than we are used to having at our disposal", and "could give us leverage in negotiating with those in control—either for better treatment of the civilians in their power (...) or for permission to provide humanitarian assistance to those populations".[37] Supporters of this view believed, however, that military operations to protect civilians were not sufficiently systematic, and overly guided by ulterior political agendas, which substantially reduced their impact.

This is why, from 1998 to 2005, MSF campaigned to get the UN and the nations participating in military operations in Bosnia and Rwanda to appoint Commissions of Inquiry, so that they could "learn lessons from these bloody failures, in order to prevent future deceptive deployments of soldiers to stand by—tied and bound—and do nothing in the face of criminal policies".[38] MSF urged the UN and Security Council members to adopt a "military doctrine on the protection of populations", making it possible to "translate it into [detailed, concrete] military actions and objectives".[39]

Another line of thought at MSF was more sceptical about criminalising and militarising the fight against mass human rights violations. As one MSF representative commented, "a Russian soldier in Chechnya, a faction head in Congo, or an American officer in Afghanistan, indeed all those who might have a concern, founded or not, that they may one day have to account for their actions in front of a court, will see in the provision of the ICC a powerful incentive to remove any humanitarian presence".[40] Especially since the prosecutor and the NGOs supporting his action called explicitly for humanitarian organisations to provide information to help him determine the appropriateness of launching an investigation and prepare the cases.[41] And coupled with this controversy was a fierce debate on the political virtues of the international criminal justice system.[42]

In the same vein, those who held this view tended to think that armed protection of civilians in conflicts was just as deadly a trap as the armed protection of aid workers. In practice, protecting populations meant occupying some or all of a country and/or toppling an oppressive regime. This involved a war operation in itself, with the attendant risk of failure, escalation, and casualties. For example, the NATO intervention in Kosovo precipitated the exodus of hundreds of thousands of Kosovars in March and April of 1999. The 40,000 soldiers deployed after the withdrawal of Serb troops over an area twice the size of a French département failed to prevent the backlash of oppression that led to the expulsion of large portions of the Serb, Bosnian and Romani minorities from the province. To those people at MSF, "calling for the military protection of a population signals the desire for a 'just war' and for the advent through violence of a new political order—and this is an undertaking that always has uncertain outcomes and which inevitably creates victims among the people it is trying to save".[43] Moreover, they maintained that MSF could not be seen as favouring armed action without endangering its access to crisis zones.

Darfur: a Return to the 1971 Charter?

So, for some at MSF, the military and punitive overtone adopted by liberal interventionism oriented it toward a repressive moralism unlikely to promote humanitarian action and human rights. Others, in contrast, saw it as a promising resource giving MSF's public statements more bite. The Darfur crisis proved that liberal interventionism could be both a resource and a liability.

Present since 2003 in the Sudanese conflict between the central government and the rebels struggling against the political and economic marginalisation of their region, MSF was able to deploy only a dozen people in Darfur in early 2004. The government, conducting an extremely murderous campaign against the insurrection's social base, was drastically limiting aid. In February 2004, MSF managed to provide very basic assistance to nearly 65,000 people, at a time when the UN placed the number of people driven from their villages by the government sponsored massacres and scorched earth policy at more than a million.

In early March 2004, MSF teams came to believe that speaking out publicly was the only way to trigger a relief operation sufficient to the needs of Darfur, and push the Sudanese government to end the most deadly and brutal aspects of its counterinsurgency strategy. But it was the UN humanitarian coordinator for Sudan who broke the silence; on 19 March 2004, he alerted the press to the severity of the violence and hardship, comparing the catastrophe in Darfur to that of Rwanda in 1994. On 7 April 2004, while the 10th anniversary of the start of the Rwandan genocide was being commemorated in Kigali, Kofi Annan urged the international community not to repeat the mistakes of Rwanda. He called upon member states to use military means if the Sudanese government continued to restrict access by humanitarian organisations and human rights investigators to Darfur.[44]

Statements by UN representatives were accompanied by a powerful public opinion campaign in the United States (just as the Abu-Ghraib prison torture scandal was erupting) demanding military intervention to put a stop to a "genocide" or a campaign of "ethnic cleansing".[45] In July 2004, Britain, Australia and Norway offered to commit troops to the UN, and in September 2004, US secretary of state Colin Powell declared that genocide had indeed been committed in Darfur, and that it might continue. At the same time, the spokesman for the Sudanese National Assembly, invoking Iraq, threatened to "open the doors of Hell"[46] should there be a foreign invasion his country. Sudanese president Omar al-Bashir maintained that "humanitarian organisations are the real enemy"[47] of Sudan.

This international pressure did, however, contribute to a significant reduction in violence and an unprecedented opening of northern Sudan to aid organisations. Beginning in the winter of 2004, more than 13,000 humanitarian workers—900 of them international—were deployed by international NGOs and UN agencies. By late 2004, MSF had more than 200 expatriate volunteers working in twenty-five projects serving some 600,000 people. In most of the camps, the mortality and malnutrition rates declined steadily, falling below the emergency threshold in early 2005. This was unprecedented in the history of the Sudanese civil war, where massacres had hitherto been followed by widespread famine.

While exposure of the crisis—and the ensuing media and diplomatic mobilisation—made such an opening possible, MSF was divided about what attitude it should take regarding the public opinion campaign for an international military intervention to "stop a genocide" in Darfur. None of the sections believed they were seeing an extermination policy comparable to that observed in Rwanda. Nevertheless, only the French section felt it necessary to distance itself from the dominant discourse then subscribed to by most NGOs.

In June 2004, the French section published the results of retrospective mortality surveys conducted in IDP camps. These were the first epidemiological field data to contradict the government's claim that there were no massacres, and showed that pro-government militias had killed several thousand people (4% to 5% of the original population of attacked villages) during the counter-insurgency campaign. But the section refuted the characterisation of genocide, questioning the existence of racial extermination doctrines and programmes in Sudan. It underscored the urgent need to expand humanitarian relief operations, now that the government had halted the most brutal aspects of its campaign, and diarrhoea and malnutrition had become the most common causes of death. The genocidal view is the result of "propagandistic distortions" wrote the president of MSF-France, condemning "certain human rights organisations" for trying to impose "a new international political order where serious human rights violations would be subject to systematic—and, if necessary, armed—international intervention".[48] In so doing, the propagandists of the genocidal view were misleading the public and the political powers about which actions were most necessary to save lives. What was needed was a massive influx of aid—not troops.

Heads of the French section believed that international military intervention aimed at occupying part of Sudan or overthrowing the regime would be a disaster, like in Iraq and Somalia, just when the level of violence had dropped sharply. MSF Holland's operations director was of the opposite opinion. Using the rhetoric developed by MSF in Bosnia, he declared that the international community would not be satisfied with an aid-only policy in Darfur. His remarks were then used by supporters of intervention, like *New York Times* columnist Nicholas Kristof, who maintained "the aid effort is sustaining victims so they can be killed with full stomachs". While the public opinion campaign condemned the rapes committed by pro-government militias as part of an "ethnic cleansing" strategy, the Dutch section published a report in March 2005 documenting over 500 cases of sexual violence and demanding that the impunity enjoyed by the perpetrators be brought to an end. A few weeks later, the Security Council took the decision to refer the Darfur crisis to the International Criminal Court. In March 2009, the ICC decided to charge Sudanese president Omar al-Bashir with war crimes and crimes against humanity. The French and Dutch sections were then expelled from Sudan, along with nine other international NGOs, accused by the government of having "violated [their] mission as humanitarian organisations" by cooperating with the "so-called International Criminal Court".[49]

The expulsion of the two MSF sections accused of collaborating with the ICC, and the rejection of the ICC by many countries where the organisation works, cast a chill over the whole movement. Since 2009, MSF has been more hesitant than ever to speak out on the crises in which it intervenes, out of fear that its words will be used to justify war or international criminal prosecutions, thus jeopardising its presence. The scepticism evidenced by some toward the international criminal justice system and armed protection for civilian populations helped to justify a policy Dr Pigeon would have agreed with—silence heals.

Some MSF members see this return to the 1971 charter as a major political step backward. They point out that without international mobilisation on Darfur, MSF would never have been able to extend its operations, and that tens of thousands of Sudanese would probably have perished from hunger and continued violence. In other words, if the United Nations hadn't broken the silence in March 2004, MSF would have had to speak out, even if that meant fuelling a political dynamic leading to the possibility of criminal or military sanctions against the Sudanese leadership. What's more, they point out, by not making a concerted effort to condemn both the regime's crimes and the propagandist lies of the neo-conservative lobbies, the entire MSF movement lost the opportunity to build political alliances beyond the western powers and the UN.

At a time when countries are more concerned than ever about their international image—to the point of codifying their intolerance of criticism in a contractual or legislative framework—MSF is reluctant to make use of its capacity to speak out. Afraid to be seen as a stakeholder in legal or military processes, and thus compromise its access to conflict zones, it tends to let other international actors speak for it, hoping to distinguish itself as the language police by tracking down misuses of humanitarian semantics. In so doing, it struggles to show its uniqueness, and to demonstrate by example the autonomy it demands.

MSF's public positions have been built on its experiences in the field, using the ideological frameworks of the moment, in the hope of strengthening and prolonging its policies for assisting populations. Influenced by neo-conservatism in the 1970s and 1980s, and then tilting toward liberal internationalism in the 1990s, MSF must now pursue its own policy based on the rejection of sacrifice[50] and ad hoc choice of its alliances. With the liberal democracies and the UN—upon whom it relied during its first thirty years—going to war, MSF is now being forced to diversify its diplomatic and political support without neglecting on principle its former comrades (e.g., UN agencies, human rights groups, western diplomacy and other humanitarian NGOs). If it wants to offer impartial, effective aid, MSF must distance itself equally from the liberal imperialism of the societies of its origins and the despotism of many of the countries where it intervenes. Experience has shown that it can only succeed with the support of political and diplomatic coalitions of convenience, rallied through an engagement in the public space, without which humanitarianism is only a passive instrument in the service of power.

Translated from French by Nina Friedman

CARING FOR HEALTH

Jean-Hervé Bradol

The first step taken by the founders of MSF was to create an organisation made up "exclusively of doctors and members of the health sector" to assist "victims of natural disasters, collective accidents and situations of belligerence".[1] At its first general assembly, they drew up a charter[2] setting forth the principles that would guide the action of the organisation. These principles of impartiality, neutrality and independence were inspired by those of the Red Cross, and later included a reference to medical ethics.

At the beginning of the 1970s, the prevailing trend among non-governmental organisations was to extend their action beyond patient medical care to health promotion. Presenting itself as an institution focusing on crisis situations and patient care therefore set MSF apart from other international aid organisations. However, its aim of providing care on the scale of a whole population was early evidence of a public health ambition. This ambition, implicit in the first version of MSF's charter (1971), was no longer so in the second version (1992), with its explicit reference to "populations in distress".

The terms "non-governmental organisation", "without borders" [sans frontières] and the "independence" of humanitarian aid workers are misleading. They imply that MSF can single-handedly decide on its objectives and the activities to be implemented to achieve them. In reality, there is no such thing as a "no man's land". However unstable a situation, any humanitarian presence, especially foreign, necessarily involves negotiations with local political and health authorities, be it the governor of a region, a health official, the officer in charge of a militia, the head of a village or a slum gang-leader. So how did MSF manage to negotiate the inclusion of a new organisation of practitioners in the public health field? This chapter does not tell the story; it is more a journey through forty years of history seen from three different angles: the discourse, the field missions and the management of the organisation's institutional development.

Contemporary public health was born in Europe and the United States in the nineteenth century during a period of social reformism and advances in knowledge on the transmission and control of infectious diseases: "Public Health[3] is the science and art of preventing disease, prolonging life and promoting physical health and efficiency through organised community efforts for the sanitation of the environment, control of community infections, educating people in personal hygiene, organisation of healthcare services for the early diagnosis and preventive treatment of disease and the development of social measures to ensure to every member of the community an adequate standard of living for the maintenance of health".[4] Dating back to the beginning of the twentieth century, this conception of public health continues to inspire health policies today.

The period we look at in this chapter (1971 to 2011) has seen major geopolitical upheavals, including decolonisation, the Cold War, the collapse of the Soviet Union, India and China's membership of the World Trade Organisation, Brazil's emergence as a global player and the extension of the European Union. As a result of these developments, public health has gradually taken on a dimension that extends beyond national frameworks, as well as those of colonial health, cooperation between two governments or regional cooperation between several states. Public health, tropical medicine, human and political sciences have all converged to create *global health*. Transnational health, a more measured expression for describing this evolution, has become a field in which institutions, public or private, local, national, regional, international or transnational, have entered into discussions, often tense, on the state of knowledge, the choice of norms, order of priorities, assessment of results and distribution of available resources.

For those operating in the field, this progression in transnational health meant determining where they stood on a series of initiatives decided within institutions such as the WHA[5] (World Health Assembly) operating on a global level. Non-governmental organisations were being asked to help governments make the major campaigns of the United Nations a reality: the Expanded Programme on Immunization (WHA, 1974), the essential medicines list (WHA, 1977), universal access to primary healthcare in 2000 (international conference on primary healthcare in Alma-Ata, 1978), the Bamako Initiative for accelerating access to primary healthcare for African populations (commitment made by African health ministers at the 37th regional meeting of the WHO, 1987), the Global Polio Eradication Initiative (AMS, 1988) and the Millennium Development Goals on health (Millennium summit, United Nations headquarters in New York, 2000).

What role should MSF play in the implementation of major public health policies? This has been the subject of debate since the organisation's first general assembly in 1972: "There are two opposing positions: the first argues for medical care to be delivered by volunteers who can be rapidly mobilised for short missions. [...] The second, supported by volunteers returning from Bangladesh and Upper Volta [now Burkina Faso], defends the principle of intervening in that other emergency: the chronic lack of medical care in the third world".[6]

At the beginning of the 1970s, this divergence was handled with pragmatism. In order to exist, and also to gain recognition, MSF's priority was to send an increasing number of doctors and nurses out to the field. This was the rationale behind its offer to second personnel to other organisations (Red Cross, UNICEF, UNHCR, Frères des Hommes, etc.), as well as to health ministries and even to the French Ministry of Cooperation, as in this project discussed in 1973: "In Yemen, the hospital would be built by the government and MSF would be responsible for running it. [...]. This type of mission could make MSF an international player. [...]. And what's more, it could be developed by young doctors on compulsory civilian service".[7]

Resisting Totalitarianism and Supporting the United Nations'
Major Campaigns

During the 1980s, MSF field missions increased. Concerns about the organisation's survival continued in an increasingly competitive environment which saw the founding of medical NGOs, such as Médecins du Monde (1980), and other bodies working in related fields, such as Action Internationale Contre la Faim (1979). MSF needed to affirm its existence, but also to distinguish itself through its presence in the field, the nature of its activities and its arguments voiced in the public arena. Meanwhile, ideological debates were gaining ground in NGOs, fuelled by political clashes in the international arena.

In the Cold War climate, the so-called under-developed countries, mainly former colonies which had recently gained independence, found themselves at the centre of a struggle for influence between the two blocs. In 1949, combating under-development was already one of the four key messages in US President Harry S. Truman's inaugural address:[8] "We must embark on a bold new programme to make the benefits of our scientific advances and industrial progress available for the improvement and growth of under-developed regions. More than half the people in the world are living in conditions approaching misery. Their food is inadequate. They are victims of disease. Their economic life is primitive and stagnant. Their poverty is a handicap and a threat both to them and to more prosperous areas". This ambition for development was shared and, to a large extent, it transcended political divisions, as had the civilising mission of colonialism in other times. But although there was consensus on the objective of development, there was also fundamental disagreement on how to achieve it: Public or private services? Economies administered by state agents or "market" agents? Capitalism or socialism?

Third-worldism, development, poor countries' debt, famine and international health issues were at the heart of the debate led by Liberté Sans Frontières (LSF), a foundation created in France by MSF (1984 to 1989). In the proceedings from the 1985 conference "Le Tiers-mondisme en question", LSF made its criticisms clear: "Basically, the tenets of the 'new order',[9] supported by the whole third world movement, have the singular characteristic of pursuing perfectly admirable objectives through means that can only lead to their failure".[10] LSF described third-worldism as the love child of "Leninism and Social Christianity", "a sort of extension of traditional social morality on a worldwide scale". These public stances were the reflection of the organisation's commitment, alongside the neo-liberals, to the various struggles underway at the end of the Cold War. So it is hardly surprising that the humanitarian doctors came out of the war in Afghanistan

(1979 to 1989) saddled with the affectionate nickname of "French doctors".

The financial issues relating to health did not escape this trend towards neo-liberal theses: "Research is a long and costly process that only pharmaceutical companies can afford, and the pharmaceutical industrialisation of the third world is no panacea".[11] These opinions were adopted at the instigation of some of MSF's management in Paris, but this marked political stance against third-worldism met with fierce and broad-based opposition among the members of the organisation in France, as well as in Belgium, where a section had been created in 1980.

As far as MSF's management team was concerned, this rejection of third-worldism was not simply ideological opposition to attempts at social and health engineering, which it perceived as being tinged with totalitarianism. The organisation's experience with assistance to refugees and its management's anti-communism fed off each other. According to the UNHCR, between 1976 and 1982, the number of refugees worldwide rose from three million to eleven million, and continued to increase until the 1990s. These refugees were Vietnamese, Cambodian, Laotian, Afghan, Ethiopian... and were proof "by their very existence of the failure of communism, as the 'people's republics' of the third world 'produced' nearly 90 per cent of the total number of the world's refugees".[12]

Missions to assist refugees were a political choice, but the camps, delimited and relatively stable, were also the perfect place for learning medical and health practices. In these camps, as a result of successive delegations (from the Ministry of Health to the UNHCR and from the UNHCR to MSF), humanitarian doctors found themselves in charge of public health. It was therefore crucial for them to shake off their image as well-intentioned, medical adventure-seekers, but ineffectual in public health terms. An image taken to heart by many humanitarian doctors, they developed an inferiority complex vis-à-vis their peers. The refugee camps in Thailand, Pakistan, Sudan, Somalia, Malawi, Rwanda, Zambia, South Africa and Honduras provided an ideal introduction to public health practices for MSF teams.

The acquisition of new expertise soon led to the compiling of clinical and therapeutic handbooks and essential medicines guidelines adapted to the specific circumstances of humanitarian medical practice. On the basis of these guidelines, medicine and medical equipment kits were put together to facilitate the launch of emergency operations and, in 1986, a logistics procurement centre was set up in France to supply the different programmes.[13] Internal training courses were organised and health managers were sent to public health schools in the United States. The intervention epidemiology developed by the CDC (Centers for Disease Control and Prevention) thus became a model for Epicentre, created in 1987, whose objective was to carry out epidemiological studies to improve the assessment of programmes and measure the results obtained in terms of public health.

The work carried out by Epicentre resulted in the drawing up of a series of priorities to be taken into account when opening a camp in an emergency situation: needs assessment, measles immunisation, water and sanitation, food, shelter, site planning and organisation, healthcare, control of communicable diseases, epidemiological surveillance, staff recruitment and training, and the coordination of operators. In this respect, the intervention in Malawi in the 1980s was viewed as the most successful refugee assistance operation: "In managing the health of almost half of the refugee population,[14] from site planning, nutrition, hygiene and public health, through to on-going epidemiological surveillance, we had to develop expertise that for the most part we only used intermittently". But there was another side to the coin. MSF personnel were busy with tasks increasingly removed from patient care. Doctors sent out to the field encountered public health for the first time and threw themselves with all the enthusiasm of novices into sanitarian campaigns with illusory outcomes, made up of authoritarian injunctions aimed at the people living in the camps.

From the early years, MSF's medical assistance to people affected by armed conflict coexisted with interventions of medical technical assistance, the aim of which was to "transfer knowledge" and help "governments set up and manage their country's health programme at national or regional level".[15] For MSF's French section, of the forty or so missions underway at the end of the 1980s, eight fell into the technical assistance category (Yemen, Madagascar, Guinea, Niger, Guatemala, Romania, Vietnam and Laos). These projects consisted of setting up immunisation programmes and primary or community healthcare programmes (water, hygiene and sanitation in the Mezquital slum in Ciudad de Guatemala). However, during the 1980s, the organisation's growing international dimension shifted the balance between missions responding to conflict situations and technical assistance.

Most of the activity (and sometimes all) of the Belgian, Swiss, Dutch and Spanish sections was, until the beginning of the 1990s, medical technical assistance.

Begun in 1981 when expatriate doctors were sent out to make up for the absence of qualified national staff in two prefectures in the north of the country, MSF-Belgium's work in Chad was a perfect example of how to support the administration of a health district, i.e. a referral hospital with a network of dispensaries. In 1983, MSF opened a pharmaceutical store to supply the hospitals and dispensaries and, by 1985, in nine prefectures of the country which had no medical school to train its own doctors, all the "préfets sanitaires", to use the country's terminology, with only one exception, were doctors sent by MSF: "De facto, Chad sub-contracted its health strategy to an NGO. From 1983, MSF had in N'Djamena an effective radio communications network, collected data, drew up epidemiological curves and planned programmes. MSF's offices were adjacent to the Ministry of Health".[16]

All these technical assistance missions followed in the wake of the major public health drives coordinated by the United Nations, in spite of Liberté Sans Frontières' reservations regarding the final declaration of the 1978 Alma-Ata conference: "Some saw it as a revolutionary text urging a radical change to society. Village health workers were presented as 'liberators' who would free their people".[17] The first criticism concerned the goal of "health for all the people of the world by 2000", which seemed to promise a totalitarian utopia: "The Conference strongly reaffirms that health [...] is a state of full physical, mental and social wellbeing, and not merely the absence of disease or infirmity". The second criticism was of the means for achieving this goal, and especially the role accorded to village health workers, modelled on the "bare-foot doctors" of Maoist China. The level of responsibility entrusted to a category of personnel with no medical or paramedical skills did not bode well for their chances of success, especially given the lack of training, supervision and material resources available to them.

In spite of these criticisms, the will to disseminate biomedical practices in countries said to be under-developed, combined with the principle of equity at the core of the primary healthcare strategy, had a unifying effect. Vaccinating children, targeting priority diseases according to their impact on mortality and the chances of treating them successfully, standardising protocols for the treatment of diseases, establishing a list of essential medicines to be supplied as generics, improving the organisation and management of healthcare facilities, all these goals seemed to be an enormous improvement on the way third world hospitals and dispensaries were usually run. The 1987 Bamako Conference had also eased some of the concerns raised by the Alma-Ata Declaration. It proposed decentralising management to health centres where care would be delivered under the supervision of qualified healthcare professionals, and suggested a means of addressing the issue of funding: users contributing towards the cost of health services. This measure was in phase with the Structural Adjustments policies of the World Bank and the International Monetary Fund that sounded the death knell of the welfare state.

MSF's overall assessment of its technical assistance activities was summed up in the report made by MSF France's president at its general assembly in 1988, a year that had been marked by financial difficulties for the organisation: "The usefulness of these missions is beyond doubt and it is very likely that in the years to come there will be extensive opportunities for funding them".[18]

The Missed Opportunities of Development and the Victory of Neo-liberalism

The growing influence of neo-liberalism at the beginning of the 1980s and its effects on health systems were not called into question by MSF at the time. Yet those of the organisation's doctors who had assumed responsibilities in public health administrations found themselves in the frontline when it came to dealing with the obstacles in implementing primary healthcare. In the wake of the Bamako Conference, these doctors had become the administrators of user contributions to the cost of health services in the hope that the revenues raised would allow access to quality care for all. But the reality was quite different: the contributions made by families could not offset the financial disengagement of the states. Anyone with insufficient means was excluded.

These budgetary tensions impacted negatively on the running of health structures and the quality of care. There was a lack of motivation amongst health staff, particularly those on the lowest salaries, sometimes resulting in high levels of absenteeism, protests, and even strikes. The adoption of new therapeutic protocols, sorely needed because bacteria and parasites were becoming increasingly resistant to usual treatments, was being hindered by budget restrictions imposed on governments.

The diversity of the health techniques required for the successful completion of these missions weighed heavily on MSF's technical support departments and the other medical, epidemiological and logistical structures established to support its operations. The recruitment department rarely found staff with the qualifications necessary to handle all the tasks at hand. In Europe, head office managers were finding it increasingly difficult to answer the questions from the field, as their own knowledge of health policies was limited. They had little contact with the two United Nations agencies, UNICEF and the World Health Organization (WHO), which were trying to coordinate the implementation of the policies.

The absence or inadequacy of biomedical practices observed over vast geographical areas, a phenomenon portrayed as the "healthcare desert", was at the origin of technical assistance missions. It pleaded in favour of a "knowledge transfer" to countries described as under-developed. However, the users showed little interest in a healthcare offer that required them to contribute in the name of "community" participation, when there had been no definition of the "community" concerned or of the healthcare expectations of the members of this so-called "community". At the end of the 1990s, an analysis of MSF activities in Guinea's Kankan prefecture clearly illustrated the limits of these types of missions: "Rapidly, the biggest problem identified by all the partners was 'low attendance rates in the dispensaries. [...] There had never been any measurement of the population's satisfaction nor of the objective parameters of morbidity or mortality. [...] Because of the cost recovery system, the sale price of drugs was partly calculated on the basis of amounts sold, and so low attendance posed a problem of financial survival for the programme".[19] For all that, did this mean giving up on technical assistance and the idea of third world development?

In 1992 criticism within MSF was no longer limited to third-worldism: the very idea that humanitarian aid should aim to contribute to development was being contested. A new definition of humanitarian action was put forward in the introduction to the first collective book to be published since Liberté Sans Frontières was made dormant in 1989: "First, let us hazard a minimum definition. Humanitarian action aims to preserve life and human dignity and to restore people's ability to choose. To accept such a definition is to say that in contrast to other areas of international solidarity, humanitarian aid does not aim to transform society but to help its members get through a crisis period, in other words when there has been a break with a previous balance".[20] This appeal to end attempts at social and health engineering also pleaded in favour of greater autonomy for MSF vis-à-vis public health policies decided by governments and the United Nations. One of the consequences of this change in position was that the organisation refocused its operations on situations of conflict and the response to epidemics and natural disasters, in tune with a new conception of humanitarian action's specific scope: emergencies. However, such interventions were too unpredictable and often too short-lived to be the only action on which to base the organisation's development. Providing assistance to refugees appeared to offer a more secure working framework, while staying within the limits set by the definition of 1992. However, this new strategy coincided with the breakup of the communist bloc, and the victory of neo-liberalism transformed perceptions of the refugee issue.

"The [Vietnamese] boat people have lost their political heft, their symbolic status and their media visibility. They are now treated on the same footing as the Albanian boat people, who were sent back to poverty by the Italian authorities, or the Haitians returned to dictatorship by the American Coast Guard in total disregard of the principles set out in the 1951 Convention on refugees. [...] The time is past when refugees testified to the superiority of democratic systems and the 'great misery' of communism".[21] The image of the dissident seeking escape, once seen as "a hymn to freedom", was replaced by that of the undesirable economic immigrant. This mutation in perception was partly due to the reticence of funding agencies, accentuated by the UNHCR's poor resource management. Host countries and funding agencies alike exerted constant pressure to ensure ever-greater reductions in aid. Any assistance to refugees was suspected of inciting economic migration.

Yet as the Cold War came to an end, civil wars in Afghanistan, Myanmar, Liberia, Somalia, Bosnia, Georgia, Sierra Leone, Burundi, Rwanda, Chechnya, etc., triggered massive exoduses, which the major powers and the United Nations attempted to contain by injecting aid into conflict zones. Internally displaced persons camps and "safe humanitarian zones" served through "humanitarian corridors" rapidly replaced camps set up beyond national borders. Yet the protection and the standard of aid received in these new camps were far inferior to that provided to refugees living in countries at peace. Repatriation, not always safe or voluntary, replaced asylum as the key word in refugee management policies.

MSF's reaction to the tensions caused by this new policy towards peoples fleeing conflict was to call for respect for their rights and compliance with health standards adopted in a geopolitical context that, since the fall of the Berlin Wall, belonged to the past. In 1989 and 1990, this shift in position led to an epidemic of pellagra among the 400,000 or so Mozambicans living in camps in Malawi.[22] Forty thousand cases of the disease were recorded, caused by dietary deficiencies, but MSF had the utmost difficulty obtaining recognition[23] of the fact that the epidemic originated from shortfalls in an aid system that didn't meet its own nutritional standards.

Learning Political Autonomy

In the middle of the 1990s, MSF's experience with technical assistance missions enabled it to recognise the need to focus attention on those excluded from primary healthcare: economic migrants, inhabitants of third world slums, unemployed people living on the streets in rich countries, low-income workers and peasants, sex workers, drug-users, under-privileged children (in orphanages and detention centres for minors or the homeless), common-law prisoners, the destitute elderly, semi-nomadic peoples, and so on. Some MSF employees on their way to work found themselves regularly stepping over people whose living conditions were so atrocious it was hard to tell whether they were still alive. Others, out for a meal in the evening, would hand a few coins to children in rags and in obviously deplorable health to keep an eye on their cars. For those who witnessed, either professionally or personally, the health of people housed in secure institutions (orphanages, prisons, detention centres for minors, hospices, asylums, etc.), the shock was even greater. Confronted with situations of distress that their actions were not addressing, getting involved in these new fields of intervention was a means of responding to the moral and political quandary in which MSF's teams found themselves. This new focus also increased the number of programmes institutional funding bodies were willing to support and contributed towards MSF's rapid growth.

The expression "new fields of intervention" implicitly referred to those programmes that did not fit into the category of aid to disaster-stricken populations (war, epidemics, natural disasters and famine) or that of technical assistance, although some of them had already been running for several years. The Mezquital slum mission in Ciudad de Guatemala and the Mission France, both opened in 1987, were prime examples.

By gradually abandoning technical assistance projects to concentrate on situations being presented as "new", MSF did not completely forsake the major United Nations campaigns, which in the meantime had evolved. In fact, the image of development had blurred to the extent that it was now suspected of exhausting the world's natural resources. As for economic growth, it had been accompanied by such an increase in social inequality that it had become difficult to believe that one day it could actually benefit the most vulnerable populations. Consequently, the United Nation's lexicon of economic and social action was updated, development policy became linked to poverty reduction, and 1996 was proclaimed international year for the eradication of poverty. In this new context, the goal was no longer "health for all the people of the world by 2000", but the partial reduction of some of the main health scourges by 2015: malnutrition, maternal, infant and child mortality, AIDS, malaria and tuberculosis. The method put forward to reach this goal relied on the combined effects of economic growth and specialised assistance programmes for the excluded, and was made up of health activities selected on the basis of a good cost-effectiveness ratio. The public health programmes promoted by the United Nations and WHO abandoned their generalist vocation to become almost exclusively specialised. Specialisation—so-called vertical programmes focusing on a delimited category of care, such as the malaria eradication programme—had existed since the beginning of the 1950s, but became systematic by the end of the 1990s.

This new policy adopted by governments and the United Nations did not garner as much support as the arguments put forward in favour of development in the 1970s. The failure of the "cost recovery" system in health centres had left its mark, especially as it was still in use. MSF's fear was of once again being associated with a policy that might backfire on its supposed beneficiaries. Rather than gamble on the hypothetical combined benefits of economic growth and assistance programmes specialised in caring for those overlooked by development, the organisation advocated for the re-inclusion of excluded populations in common-law health systems. For MSF, this didn't mean simply demanding the enforcement of existing rights, but formulating new ones and promoting their incorporation in national and international legislation. Thus, in France the organisation was not only active in drafting the law on universal health coverage but battled over each and every point of the decree.

In the case of MSF's programme in Madagascar, which provided medical treatment to "street children", aspirations for the government to assume its role became so intense that it led to its closure in 2005, despite the ever-increasing number of people excluded from healthcare with no public services lined up to replace it: "Today, 70% of the capital's inhabitants live below the poverty line. There is less and less difference between homeless families living in the street and everybody else. [...] Yet the issue of medical treatment and healthcare for the poor is a political, economic and social one, and should be addressed by the public authorities. Poverty reduction is today's goal. [...] A humanitarian organisation such as MSF has neither the mandate nor the ability to replace the authorities and provide access to healthcare for all of a town's impoverished population".[24] But the fact remains that even if the cooperation with the health ministries had not always helped improve access to healthcare for the least well-off, breaking it off completely was going to cause further hardship.

The Response to Epidemics and Immersion in Global Health

Is it possible to oppose public policies that are detrimental to patient care without becoming isolated and giving up on trying to influence them? A public health action on a global scale—the relaunch of the combat against infectious diseases—gave MSF the opportunity to explore different avenues to answer this question. The renewed interest of governments and international organisations in infectious diseases was triggered by a prognosis made in 1992 by the National Academy of Science in the United States, which presented infectious diseases as a threat to health likely to "persist and even intensify in the future".[25] In 1995, the WHO set up a division headed by a director recruited from the CDC for the surveillance and control of emerging and communicable diseases.

MSF had been involved in responses to epidemics and major endemics, both in refugee camps and in so-called open environments, for more than fifteen years as part of its technical assistance. Programmes aimed at controlling sleeping sickness had begun in Moyo, Uganda in

1986 and since the beginning of the 1980s, interventions in the camps had brought the teams up against a wide range of epidemics: cholera, measles, meningitis, shigellosis, etc.

In 1995, MSF helped to relaunch the combat against infectious diseases, partly to address real needs on the ground and partly to offset the reduction in technical assistance projects and programmes in refugee camps. At the beginning of 1996 MSF ran a meningitis immunisation campaign in the northern states of Nigeria: almost three million people were vaccinated and thirty thousand patients were treated for the infection.

The emergence of new epidemics (Ebola and AIDS, in particular), the re-emergence of old diseases (such as tuberculosis and hemorrhagic dengue), and the fear of bioterrorism (rekindled by a handful of anthrax letter attacks in some big North American cities in 2001), prompted governments to take action. In 2000, in a report that has since become famous,[26] the CIA confirmed that the issue was being taken very seriously as "infectious diseases posed a threat to national security, the economy and political stability". The concern, not necessarily justified from an epidemiological point of view, was provoked mainly by the progression of epidemics due to HIV. Resolution 1308 of the United Nations Security Council in 2000 "stress[ed] that the HIV/AIDS pandemic, if unchecked, may pose a risk to stability and security". The World Bank described AIDS as the "crisis of development". In September 2000, the United Nations General Assembly adopted the Millennium Declaration, with one of its goals formulated as follows: "to have [...] halted, and begun to reverse, the spread of HIV/AIDS, the scourge of malaria and other major diseases that afflict humanity" by the year 2015.

For international organisations and governments providing the funding for this goal, the programme that eradicated smallpox in 1979 was an ideal model for combating infectious diseases. Based on preventing new cases by containing transmission to such an extent that the disease disappeared, it required an initial investment of several years (the immunisation campaign) and resulted in a conclusive outcome (the elimination of the disease).

Three conditions are required for implementing such a strategy: effectiveness, price and universal availability. Yet the cost of new medical products prior to large-scale use is always prohibitive for public health institutions and users. They can only be widely prescribed once specific economic models are developed for the launch of major public health actions.

But there is a further constraint specific to drugs for treating infections. Treatments must be renewed rapidly because bacteria, parasites and viruses develop resistances at a fast rate. In infectiology, practitioners usually need recent and expensive drugs. Yet at the end of the 1990s, the situation had deteriorated to such an extent that even the old but still effective medicines were beginning to run out. At the international medical symposium on the response to epidemics organised by MSF in 1996,[27] participants pointed to a lack of research: among the 1,000 new molecules put on the market since 1975 only ten or so had been developed for the treatment of tropical diseases and tuberculosis.[28] As a result, in the middle of the 1990s, medicines—whether for treating epidemics (AIDS, meningitis, etc.), major endemics (tuberculosis, sleeping sickness) or banal community infections (pneumonia, malaria, etc.)—were in increasingly short supply. The response by governments and international organisations to malaria (insecticides and mosquito nets) and AIDS (drive to change sexual behaviour and promote use of condoms) focused exclusively on preventive measures. Treatment for tuberculosis was concentrated on patients who had the bacteria in their sputum and could therefore contaminate their entourage. There was a clear gap between the offer (the medical products available) and the demand (clinical and health priorities in infectiology). Practitioners working in countries where infectious diseases were still the primary cause of mortality gradually found themselves without the means to take effective action.

At the beginning of the 2000s, a multitude of institutions (national public administrations, international organisations, pharmaceutical companies, private national and international associations, religious institutions, trade unions, political parties, etc.) endeavoured to improve this situation of penury. The internet was the preferred vector for relations that transcended borders, evolved and reached out to the most peripheral stakeholders (patients, care providers, citizens) and the summits of health institutions (WHO, UNICEF, etc.), economic institutions (World Trade Organization, WTO), and political institutions (United Nations General Assembly and Security Council, G8). Until then, questions concerning access to medicines had been discussed behind closed doors and the only participants were experts, industrialists and state representatives. Now, the debate on conditions of access to new medicines had become the object of considerable media attention and the presence of AIDS-response organisations and practitioners such as MSF at the negotiating table was deemed necessary.

Remembering the lessons learnt from its experience with medical technical assistance, MSF created the Campaign for Access to Essential Medicines, financed in part by the Nobel Peace Prize that it had been awarded in 1999. It was important to avoid finding itself once again being associated with a transnational public health campaign without having any influence over the decisions taken at the top, whether at national level in the ministries of health or within international organisations such as the WHO. MSF urged that the fight against infectious diseases should not be based exclusively on preventive measures to eradicate the pathogenic agents, but that it should also include treatment for those suffering from them. To this end, new medical products would be needed and their use incorporated into national and international strategies.

At the end of the 1990s, MSF decided that to influence public policies action was required at the very root of the problem. This meant identifying levers to secure changes in policy and establish new alliances. So MSF developed links with activist organisations such as South Africa's Treatment Action Campaign and countries such as Brazil and Thailand, which were striving to broaden access to medicines protected by patents in middle-income countries. MSF was now represented at every link in the chain: at the patient's bedside, at meetings in hospitals, in the office of the physician in charge of health at district or regional level, at the ministry, at the offices of international organisations, at scientific congresses, whenever and wherever international activists were organised (the G8 counter-summits, for example), but also in the offices of the heads of states' sherpas, at the headquarters and factories of pharmaceutical companies, in the administrative departments responsible for importing medical products—and of course in the public debate.[29]

Why was it that in the case of AIDS, for example, the national governments providing the funding agreed to derogate from the "smallpox elimination" model and undertook to spend several billion euros annually in treating millions of patients, in spite of the fact that there was little prospect of the disease being eliminated? A partial explanation for this untypical behaviour is to be found in the threat AIDS poses to public security, the exceptional level of social mobilisation, the fear of serious economic fallout and the rapid scientific advances. It was also essential to take into account the importance of public debate on the issue of intellectual property rights and the pharmaceuticals trade.

At the end of the 1990s, the WTO focused on the globalisation of the rules on intellectual property rights applicable to trade. But the commercial monopoly granted to pharmaceutical laboratories depositing a patent was largely responsible for the high price of new treatments, especially antiretrovirals. A public health disaster coupled with the prohibitive cost of medicines (several thousand dollars per year and per patient) raised the question of the compatibility of intellectual property rules with public security and, notably, health. The stakes were high: the tension between the two imperatives, respect for private property and public security, was weakening the economic system. It thus became urgent for the United States, the European Union and Japan, the main promoters of the new rules on intellectual property, to make a number of concessions on access to medicines. Their attitude of indifference, aggressiveness even, shared by the major pharmaceutical multinationals, was in danger of triggering a strong reaction against the extension of intellectual property rules to world trade as a whole. Thus, a few months before the WTO Ministerial Conference in Doha (2001), and against the backdrop of the Pretoria court case,[30] United States trade representative Robert B. Zoellick appealed to the pharmaceutical companies to see reason: "If they don't get ahead of this issue, the hostility that generates could put at risk the whole intellectual property rights system".[31] In the wake of his appeal, the major economic powers meeting at the Doha Conference agreed to moderate their stance on the enforcement of intellectual property rights in the strict domain of the pharmaceuticals trade with public health institutions. As a result, tritherapies against HIV appeared on the market in the form of generics and in fixed-dose combinations: their price fell to below 100 dollars per year, per patient. More than five million patients in low- or middle-income countries are now receiving this treatment.

The struggle against AIDS has benefited from exceptional economic and political circumstances. Indeed, to develop the political autonomy of humanitarian medicine it is essential to recognise, and sometimes anticipate, the appearance of such favourable circumstances, as this is when the most rapid and profound changes to public health policies can be achieved. Such circumstances can be neither permanent nor artificially induced through advocacy.

In such times, a breach in the political space opens up and offers an opportunity to reshape social relations, some of which may have been frozen for years. This is then an ideal opportunity to attempt to reduce the number of deaths, the suffering and the frequency of incapacitating handicaps within groups of people who are usually poorly served by public health systems. In view of the huge health gaps prevailing in large communities, the impact of humanitarian medical action is not to be restricted to the specific needs of marginal groups. Take the example of AIDS: the care protocol developed by humanitarian doctors has made it possible to treat millions of infected people throughout the world. This protocol is characterised by the non-participation of patients in the cost of tritherapies, the prescription of generic antiretrovirals combined into a single tablet, as few laboratory tests as possible, the transfer of therapeutic information and responsibilities to patients and a member of their entourage, and the participation of paramedics in the prescription.

Humanitarian medicine is not a marginal practice on the fringes of biomedicine and public health; it is an attempt to respond to the expectations of those people who are deprived of access to healthcare, in spite of their sometimes considerable demographic weight. Its specific and most important contribution to public health consists in developing medical practices that are better adapted to the living conditions and priorities of patients who are generally ignored. So not only must it constantly renew its own practices, but also, in order to prove the effectiveness of these practices, publish the results and comply with the standards of biomedicine and evidence-based medicine. However, political decision and scientific certitude operate on different timescales. Supporting or contesting a public health policy means daring to hope for a change that may not happen.

There are many examples of humanitarian medical action becoming more effective when it allows patients supported by their families more autonomy and establishes a less asymmetrical relationship with them. The implementation of HIV treatment programmes therefore provided an opportunity to change old habits with regard to the sharing of responsibilities between patients, their entourage and the medical team, and between the medics and paramedics on the care team. In another domain, the introduction of new products to treat malnutrition in young children has been extremely instructive:[32] the success of this innovation is due in part to improvements in the composition of therapeutic foods, but ultimately to the fact that these foods respond to requests from mothers who want to be able to treat their children at home as simply as possible. This suggests that, in order to better draw up the terms of its relationship with patients and the people around them, humanitarian medicine should pay heed to social sciences, and especially to schools of thought that, like the theories of care,[33] offer a new perception of the relationship between the person cared for and the care provider.

However, demonstrating the superiority of a therapeutic protocol through a few innovative programmes is not enough to ensure its integration in public health policy. The emergence of a new economic model that supports innovation is essential for it to be disseminated at public health level, and this means forming political and economic alliances. The attitude of national governments, international organisations and private companies and foundations towards finding solutions to public health crises is critical, as it can have grave consequences on the way these evolve. The political aspect of the humanitarian operator's work therefore first consists in exposing this responsibility by offering tangible proof that it is possible to do better. But dissidence is quickly replaced by the search for consensus on the reforms of care protocols. Consequently, the humanitarian doctor is a political ally who is neither stable nor faithful: sometimes dissident, sometimes consensual. The political autonomy of humanitarian medicine is founded on the mobility of its alliances.

NATURAL DISASTERS

"DO SOMETHING!"

Rony Brauman, interviewed by Claudine Vidal

> Has MSF always considered natural disasters part of its mission?

Alongside armed conflicts, natural disasters are the first category of intervention to be cited by the authors of MSF's charter and by-laws. Moreover, among the events that led to the founding of MSF were the earthquake in Peru that killed 30,000 people in May 1970, and the Bhola cyclone that hit eastern Pakistan in November in the same year, leaving 250,000 to 500,000 people dead. Natural disasters have always taken centre stage for the organisation. If you remember, MSF was formed through the merger of two associations created in 1970: GIMCU (Groupe d'intervention médico-chirurgicale d'urgence—Group for Medical and Surgical Emergency Intervention), founded by former Red Cross volunteers in Biafra, and SMF (Secours médical français—French Medical Relief), set up by medical journal *Tonus* to respond to the disaster in eastern Pakistan. This was the time when emergency medicine was gaining momentum as a specific category of care and "collective accidents", as they were curiously named in the charter, were the ideal field in which to practise it.

But GIMCU's first experience in a disaster situation, Peru in 1970, was a failure: the French doctors arrived on the scene a week after the earthquake and, in spite of the scale of the disaster, didn't encounter a single injured person. What they did find was that the countries in the region, including the United States, had already delivered emergency relief.

The lesson learnt from this first attempt at emergency intervention held sway for a long time and became a principle for all earthquakes: to implement a life-saving operation in such situations, medical assistance had to come on stream within the first forty-eight hours. Any later and the victims trapped under rubble, the injured suffering from multiple trauma—with or without crush syndrome—would have no chance of survival. So, MSF focused from the outset on reducing deployment time by ensuring emergency supplies ("kits") were ready and waiting, and doing its utmost to get its teams out to the disaster area within twenty-four hours of the alert. But to no avail. It wasn't until 2005 and the earthquake in Pakistan's Kashmir that we actually operated on casualties for the first time—although we weren't on site and operational immediately.

Earthquakes and other disasters have become more frequent in recent years. According to the CRED (Centre for Research on the Epidemiology of Disasters), the yearly average number of earthquakes causing more than ten fatalities increased from twenty-one between 1960 and 1990 to thirty at the beginning of the twenty-first century, with peaks recorded in 1990, 2003 and 2004. But only a few led to an international relief operation. In fact, we only respond to large earthquakes, when the initial estimate of fatalities is in the thousands and the national authorities call for international assistance. This is a useful reminder to us that, in spite of this type of disaster's high rank in the hierarchy of emergency humanitarian assistance, MSF had had very little experience in the field until the beginning of the new millennium. Furthermore, as over 80% of earthquakes occur in the "Pacific Ring", the distance from Europe makes the objective dictated by the precepts of emergency medical assistance of getting to the disaster site within forty-eight hours totally unrealistic. But distance and time to deploy do not explain everything, as we saw in 1990 when an earthquake leaving 37,000 dead hit Zandjan in Iran. MSF's medico-surgical teams were on site twenty-six hours later, but as their sole medical activity was providing routine consultations and totally unrelated to the traumatology they were expecting, ten days later they packed their bags and left.

It took us some time to realise that earthquakes didn't lead to a particularly high number of casualties, and that most of these received immediate treatment in local health facilities around the disaster area. Foreign medical teams, unless they were already on site, were in fact superfluous to requirement. Earthquakes were far from providing the situation par excellence that we had imagined for exercising emergency medicine, in spite of breathtaking figures evoking thousands, or even tens of thousands of casualties. However, given the symbolic importance of natural disasters in emergency assistance, it was almost inconceivable for an organisation claiming emergency response as its culture and expertise not to be part of the action. So, at the beginning of the 1990s, MSF changed direction and focused on its other skill, logistics, securing the supply of drinking water, for example, and when necessary setting up medical consultations in the places where the victims were assembled. The images of numerous surgical teams rushed off their feet and operating non-stop that we have witnessed since the earthquake in Port-au-Prince are so close to conventional representations of disaster medicine that we tend to forget that they are, in fact, relatively new, as they were seen for the first time in Kashmir in 2005.

> What happened in Kashmir in October 2005? Did the relief operations launched in response to this disaster differ from previous experience?

When news of the earthquake reached us, MSF-France's operations managers were initially extremely reluctant to intervene, for all the reasons I've just mentioned. But MSF-Belgium and MSF-Holland were in the country at the time and their teams were reporting back to us on the enormity of the disaster and particularly on the huge number of casualties. The province's health facilities were all completely overwhelmed. According to official estimates, there were tens of thousands of critically and seriously injured people in need of orthopaedic and intensive medical care. However accurate these figures, and I'll come back to this point later, it was clear that for the first time in an emergency situation the local facilities were submerged by the inflow of polytraumatised patients and unable to cope.

I think the explanation behind this sudden increase in the number of injured is the trend towards urbanisation, in other words, the densification of badly built dwellings in a high-risk seismic region. In Kashmir, people were no longer living in shantytowns, but in unsound houses made of poorly cemented breezeblocks and stones. While partial collapse of this type of construction results in crushed limbs, the victims are not buried under rubble, as they would be in buildings with several floors. But shantytowns at least have an advantage in that the wooden, plastic or sheet metal partitions used to build them cause little damage when they collapse. A reminder that all that is "natural" in a disaster is what causes it, i.e. the origin of the seismic or climatic event. Whereas the aftermath is the result of decisions made by people, such as the location or construction standards or insufficiently protected industrial installations in hazard zones. To return to the situation in Kashmir, urban densification was not simply the result of the rural exodus common to all countries, but was also part of a deliberate population distribution strategy linked to separatist intrigues and the ongoing territorial dispute with India since partition in 1947. Nonetheless, for the first time in the history of emergency responses to an earthquake, international medical and surgical teams had a real and major role.

> In 2005, the press reported that access to the victims was often impossible. What practical solutions were found to overcome this?

Access to the region was indeed difficult at first because of its geography, but also because of its politics. Kashmir is a sloping plateau in the east and is easily accessible from India. But, on the Pakistani side, there is a barrier of escarpments which is difficult to cross. Landslides stopped us from using the roads and as it was early winter, poor weather conditions further complicated matters. We had to use helicopters, which are great for transporting personnel, but their low cargo capacity meant they were not suitable for a disaster of such magnitude. These practical difficulties were the main problems we encountered, if we don't count the initial resistance of the Pakistani army, whose main concern at that point was to provide assistance to its own troops and maintain control over a province of strategic importance in its dispute with India.

The physical obstacles could have been overcome by bringing aid in via India, and the Indian government did indeed offer assistance to

Pakistan. But such an offer was unacceptable to the Pakistani army, which refused it outright, although it did agree to a partial opening of the border. This doesn't mean, however, that the army only concerned itself with its own personnel and territorial security, leaving the population without assistance. On the contrary, after a few days, it did more and more, bringing in aid supplies, treating and evacuating the injured by helicopter, and managing the coordination of the relief operations. Restrictions on movements were lifted and special permits were no longer required to travel around the tribal areas.

A multitude of local NGOs quickly got down to work, helping the victims get organised in collective centres and providing shelters. Some had highly competent personnel and were particularly well-equipped— in particular, the Al Rasheed Trust. An Islamic organisation ideologically close to the Pakistani Taliban, it set up a sixty-bed hospital for orthopaedic surgery and ran outreach and relief activities. Our collaboration with the army, the Health Ministry and Al Rasheed was excellent on the whole, much to the surprise of MSF's management staff, who had expected things to be more complicated. The local Islamic organisations, which benefit from well-established social aid networks, took immediate action and supplied a considerable amount of aid.

Let's not lose sight of the fact that most of the search for survivors and provision of food and shelter in the early stages of any disaster situation are always handled by local people and organisations. Contrary to conventional belief, it isn't a state of shock that we witness but rather active solidarity, at least during the first few weeks. So, although there was nothing surprising about the extent of local mobilisation in Kashmir, it needs to be said that once they had seen that MSF wasn't involved in any proselytising and that patients were being properly cared for, the Islamic NGOs were particularly cooperative. Islamic organisation members even praised the invaluable logistical assistance it had received from the American army.

The situation was one of close cooperation with the Ministry of Health, the army—whose helicopters we even used on occasion—and religious NGOs. Our constructive relationship with our natural partners, the health authorities and the Pakistani NGOs, raised no issues for MSF. However, despite the crucial role it played, as we have seen, the same could not be said of the army, viewed by MSF as a compromising partner. Some of the MSF operational leaders even suggested trimming down the teams in order to limit contact. This determination

to reassert the distinction between military and humanitarian operators, motivated by concerns for the teams' safety, ended up taking a
back seat to imperatives for urgent action in a context marked by the
ongoing emergency and the otherwise fruitful working relations with
all the different actors, whatever conflicts may have opposed them in
the past.

In situations of natural disaster, the national army is usually the best
placed and the best equipped to respond and, apart from exceptional
cases (such as in the zone controlled by the LTTE in Sri Lanka after the
2004 tsunami), is welcomed by the victims. So there is no reason to
actively distance ourselves, as we rightly do in situations of conflict.
This applies equally to medical relief and logistics provided by foreign
armed forces.

Taking into account the material difficulties caused by the geography of the area, the deployment of the aid operation was dynamic and,
within three weeks, had reached a level where the needs were being
met. However, when it came to medical care MSF's teams noted that,
whereas the country's response had been rapid and profuse, standards
were not so satisfactory: amputations were numerous, probably overly
so, and already conservative orthopaedic interventions—for saving
injured limbs—were often below par. Let's keep in mind that most of
the surgery performed by MSF's teams, who had not dealt with the initial influx of casualties, consisted in secondary surgery. However, I
should point out that any reservations regarding the quality of the
medical treatment stem from clinical impressions rather than from the
findings of epidemiological studies, and that this was a context of
damage-control surgery in the face of a very high number of wounded
patients.

But overwhelmed medical facilities do not explain everything. In my
opinion, we should also examine why war surgery techniques were
used. Penetrating wounds caused by projectiles (bullets, shrapnel, etc.)
can lead to complications, notably infections, which, in the uncertain
environment of an armed conflict, may prompt the surgeon to perform
more radical surgery. But wounds caused by crushing, the common lot
of civilian surgery, permit the use of more conservative techniques. Yet,
as we saw in Indonesia during the 2004 tsunami and again after the
Haiti earthquake in 2010, the paradigm of war, or in this case a blitz-
krieg, always seems to prevail. The medical teams are just as much
influenced by this representation as the observers, as revealed by a

remark made by a team of American relief workers: "Overworked surgeons [...] amputated limbs and debrided infected tissue. [...] For the next two days, we practiced continuous battlefield medicine".[1] We are justified in asking ourselves if this kind of representation has an impact on the techniques used, and studies are being conducted using medical data collected in Haiti, the only other natural disaster, along with the one in Kashmir, to have caused such massive numbers of casualties.[2] The very recent experience of mass surgery in such circumstances explains the current lack of systematised knowledge on the subject.

We also lack reliable quantitative data to draw up a comprehensive evaluation of the relief operation in Pakistan. The figures provided the day after the disaster—54,000 dead, 77,000 injured and hundreds of thousands made homeless—give an indication of the scale of the catastrophe, but should be viewed with caution, particularly from a medical standpoint. In the light of the absence of civilian registration and demographic data, the number of fatalities can only be a rough estimate.

The civil-military cooperation—read "military leadership" of the relief operations—was hailed as a success by the United Nations and the NGOs. The dividing up into sector-based groups of responsibility or "clusters" (logistics, health, sanitation, etc.), which the army had less trouble adapting to than the humanitarian operators (as was noted with some irony by the United Nations representative),[3] was also a success.

However, de facto truces resulting from a natural disaster do not signal an end to hostilities, and we mustn't lose sight of the political or even counter-insurrectional dimension of aid. The extremely sensitive deployment of US and NATO forces in response to the earthquake was explicitly dictated by such considerations. It encountered no visible opposition, as all the population was concerned with what was provided and not with who was providing it. As for the Islamic groups, they mostly kept silent, although some of them did express their approval publically. A study conducted by the US Institute for Peace concludes that the objective of "winning hearts and minds" remained theoretical, for the activist groups and for the United States and NATO, as momentary gratitude does not lead to political loyalty. But as this belief tends to hold sway, it results in more latitude for action, as nobody wants to be seen as the one depriving the people of valuable aid during a period of acute crisis.

> What is your definition of a natural disaster?

A disaster disrupts the ordinary course of things. From the purely practical standpoint of an emergency medical organisation, this first means
earthquakes and then severe climatic events—storms, cyclones and
flooding—occurring in or close to densely populated areas. Earthquakes have been our sole topic of conversation so far, as they have
recently become the main cause of emergency medical operations. But
looking at things from a broader angle, and to use more commonly
accepted definitions, a disaster can be defined as a sudden encounter
between natural forces of harm and a people in harm's way, where
demands exceed the disaster-affected community's capacity to cope or,
in other words, it is "the product of the encounter between hazards
and vulnerability".[4]

The problem with these definitions resides in the definition of "natural". The causal event may be natural, but the aftermath is closely
linked to the way society is organised in the places where they occur.
For example, you may remember that in Ethiopia (1985) and Niger
(2005), the drought and the ensuing invasion of locusts were described
by the authorities as a "natural disaster", and the primary cause of a
situation of acute malnutrition or famine. The stakes were high
because attributing these consequences to this cause determined the
response. MSF was expelled from both countries after a political controversy on these issues.[5] Remember the ironically evocative titles of
the two books published by the organisation on the subject: *Ethiopie.
Du bon usage de la famine* [*Ethiopia: How to make best use of a famine*], and *A Not-So Natural Disaster, Niger 2005.*[6]

The cholera outbreak in Haiti during the winter of 2010 to 2011 was
the source of an intense controversy of the same nature: the advocates
of a "natural" hypothesis attributed its origin to plankton and opposed
all those who claimed that the infestation was of human origin (caused
by the emptying of a septic tank containing cholera germs into a river).
Everyone agreed that the disease had only been able to result in so
many fatalities (4,800 in total) because of the country's deplorable
hygiene conditions, but the circumstances that led to the outbreak were
the subject of virulent dissension, even within MSF. The fact that the
human origin was blamed on a contingent of United Nations peace-
keepers, themselves embroiled in political clashes as a result of the election campaign underway at the time, only served to accentuate the
political dimension of the epidemic. As it happens, an enquiry con-

ducted by the United Nations later confirmed the second hypothesis.[7] Once again, it was not simply a matter of determining the origin of the epidemic; understanding its cause had practical consequences on how the immediate medico-sanitary response was organised.

> The controversies seem to be as much due to the definition of natural disasters as to the evaluation of their consequences?

As we have just seen, the rebranding of a situation from major crisis to natural disaster can lead to controversy because of the political responsibilities that such a categorisation engages. But independent of any disagreement on this aspect, the consequences of a disaster can also be a source of controversy, particularly (but not exclusively), with regard to the epidemics they might cause, and hence the emergency resources that should be deployed. Because of the unprecedented media attention it attracted, the 2004 tsunami saw this question propelled into the public arena.

A few days after this exceptionally large-scale disaster, the WHO's operations director announced: "We may see as many fatalities from disease as from the actual disaster itself".[8] So the subject was raised of a possible second wave of mortality due to epidemics, which threatened to double the number of victims caused by the actual tsunami. It was brought up by the WHO at subsequent press conferences and passed on enthusiastically by the media, with the result that the relief effort focused on providing emergency assistance to save some 150,000 people supposedly in danger of imminent death. The success of such announcements, without scientific or empirical basis, stems from how well they fit in with the widespread belief that decomposing bodies are a source of infectious contamination. Yet as several research studies have shown, there have been no cases of a fatal epidemic in the wake of a disaster, whatever the scale.[9] Put quite simply, epidemics cause corpses, but corpses don't cause epidemics. Some epidemic foci of digestive and respiratory infections may occur and require preventive and curative action, but their effects are nothing like the scaremongering announcements I just mentioned.

More generally, and for reasons similar to those I talked about earlier in relation to earthquakes, there was no life-and-death emergency after the tsunami. The horrendous ordeal suffered by a large number of survivors, some of whom lost everything, justified in itself the appeal for solidarity, and I'm certainly not disputing the need to respond to it. But the model adopted of "rescuing a population in peril" was totally inappropriate. At one point, we saw up to twelve surgeons gathered around just one casualty in Indonesia, right when we were talking in terms of hundreds of thousands of casualties! In practice, to be of real help to the victims of the disaster, the need was for financial and material resources to clear up and start rebuilding—quite different from launching an emergency medical operation. However, media pressure was such that it made it difficult for MSF to stay away. The field teams lost no time in raising the issue; some of the most experienced members had grasped what was happening within a few days. But withdrawing from the country would not have been understood in a situation so emotionally-charged, and the organisation's leadership decided to switch the focus to non-medical aid.

> Can the way a disaster is presented after the event make a difference then?

As we've seen, the scale of mobilisation shrank all the narrations, beliefs and prevailing representations of the event. Talk was of casualties, refugees, epidemics and, when UNICEF issued a statement, orphans too. We have already discussed casualties and epidemics, but the issue of refugees and orphans was much the same. I'll say more about this in a moment, but first I want to emphasise that these four themes, recurrent during the first few weeks, formed a narration of the consequences usually observed in armed conflicts. In other words, with the benefit of a little hindsight, it becomes clear that we were unconsciously reacting to a natural disaster as if it were a war.

There were endless pictures and non-stop television images of the after-effects of the disaster, focusing on a few hundred people assembled in makeshift shelters, "showing" the existence of refugee camps, whereas, in reality, people were not gathering, but rather dispersing. Most of them wanted to stay as close to their homes as possible and were living with neighbours or family and moving back and forth between their former homes and their temporary accommodation. The same goes for the destruction caused by the tsunami. In Sri Lanka, for example (except in the hardest hit region in the north), it was concentrated along a narrow strip of land between 50–300 metres wide, depending on the lay of the land where the wave hit. So the survivors were in fact only a few minutes' walk at most from the unaffected parts of the country, something we couldn't tell from the pictures we were seeing. This kind of metonymical representation, of which aid workers are as guilty as journalists, is seriously misleading. I should also add that the thousands of Sri Lankan doctors and nurses, who arrived within hours to help their colleagues and fellow citizens, were no more visible as they were indistinguishable from the disaster victims. These misinterpretations were given such credence because they fit in so well with the preconceived notion mentioned earlier of disaster victims in a state of total shock, passively waiting for help to arrive.

As for the orphans described by the director of UNICEF as wandering the streets at the mercy of child prostitution gangs, this was a rumour spread all too hastily, but rapidly dissipated by other humanitarian organisations, and by UNICEF itself. Obviously there is no question that some children had lost their parents, but what I do contest is that they had been abandoned. I should perhaps explain at this point that the post-tsunami solidarity movement, often portrayed in the North as exemplary and cited as a reference, in fact left the concerned countries with memories of an agitated, arrogant and ineffectual mob. Despite its endeavours to distance itself from the prevailing discourse, MSF did not escape from harsh collective judgement.

But let me return for a moment to the schema of war superimposed on that of natural disaster. In spite of images that make them look very similar, they are in fact diametrically opposed. Disasters are concentrated into a very limited time period and a very restricted geographical area, whereas armed conflicts are spread over an extended time period and wide geographical area. Wars are drawn out affairs, erratic in their movements, killing and injuring in their path, causing the displacement and re-assembly of populations between one region and another, creating intense and relentless pressure, rampant and massive impoverishment and wide-spread destruction, including of health facilities. These vulnerability factors, producing all these effects and creating a high potential for epidemics, cannot be caused by a one-off event. A natural disaster, however horrendous, cannot engender the same consequences as a war.

> Is there a clear association between the myths surrounding events after a disaster and political situations?

International emergency aid is loaded with a specific kind of symbolism that has nothing to do with its real usefulness, as we have just seen.

It is inevitably an intrinsic part of the pre-existing dynamics of international relations—and becomes an extension of them. For example, when Iran was hit by an earthquake in June 1990, the French government offered to send in specialised teams, even though the two countries had broken off diplomatic relations: the emergency aid brought to light the fact that Paris and Teheran had secretly resumed talks. The same can be said of China sending a plane full of aid supplies to Haiti after the earthquake in January 2010, in spite of the absence of diplomatic relations between the two countries owing to Haiti's recognition of Taiwan. This was a first. Beijing had never before contributed towards disaster relief operations outside its regional sphere of influence in Asia. However, the fact that China now wants to assert its status as a global power meant taking part in the international relief effort. Just as the earthquake in Pakistan proved the existence of a "disaster policy", there is also "disaster diplomacy", whereby the special circumstances created by an emergency allow governments to demonstrate their strategic choices at little cost.

In this respect, the case of Cyclone Nargis, which hit Myanmar in 2008, merits attention. In May 2008, the Irrawaddy delta was swept by winds reaching 240 km per hour, followed by a wave four to six metres high, which surged up the river resulting in extensive loss of life and massive destruction in this densely populated and fertile region. The Myanmar junta, faithful to its obsession with maintaining order and as ever indifferent to the fate of its people, did not react, simply appealing to the United Nations for international aid and refusing any new foreign presence on its soil. However, right from the first few days, members of MSF and other NGOs already working in the country were able to travel to the area, assess the extent of the damage and launch the relief effort with the local resources at hand. At the same time, planes from neighbouring India, Thailand, Bangladesh and Malaysia, as well as from western counties acting on behalf of UN agencies, were landing in the capital city, Yangon. In the meantime, the press and western governments, apparently unable to see beyond the junta's sovereigntist and isolationist rhetoric, were talking about restrictions and even a total blockade of outside aid. On 11 May, the NGO Oxfam issued a communiqué and the first few lines set the tone: "International agency Oxfam said today (11 May) that in the coming weeks and months the lives of up to 1.5 million people are in danger in the Myanmar cyclone zone because of the risk of disease and a public health catastrophe if clean water and sanitation are not urgently provided".

Seen from the field, this scaremongering was far from justified. It was true that the army had been seen diverting aid for its own purposes or to make a profit out of distributing it but, as always, the population got itself organised on different levels. Local organisations and authorities, the Red Cross, Buddhist temples and wealthy businessmen all distributed water, food and equipment, and foreign aid began arriving via the NGOs. As for the injured and the threats of epidemic, I repeat what I said earlier about the tsunami; they were non-existent.

It was striking that most of the television coverage, whether videos made by local people or official television reports, all showed scenes of aid distribution almost everywhere. We saw endless short scenes of businessmen arriving with their lorries and handing out bottles of water, sacks of rice, etc. Elsewhere, Buddhist monks were similarly shown, as was the army, an NGO or the Myanmar Red Cross. Basically, we were seeing the usual images of food distribution and, here and there, one or two bodies. Watching the media coverage attentively, I realised that the commentaries accompanying the pictures were actually contradicting everything they were showing, insisting on the total absence of aid and the numbers of decomposing bodies, which were described as bacteriological time bombs on the brink of spreading their deadly emanations. When I asked some journalists during interviews on the subject what they thought about the dissonance between the pictures and the commentary, they said they hadn't noticed it and were obviously suspicious of any challenge to the general alarmist view.

So it was in this context that threats of military intervention to impose aid by force first began to appear in the press. Gareth Evans, one of the authors of the UN's "Responsibility to protect" concept, started the ball rolling on 12 May,[10] followed two days later by Robert Kaplan, one of the most prominent neo-conservative strategists, who sketched the outline for armed intervention in an article entitled, "Aid at the Point of a Gun".[11] And on 19 May, French foreign minister Bernard Kouchner published an article reminding us that "the Security Council can at any time decide to intervene to force a passage for humanitarian aid, as has been done in the past".[12] Three military vessels, British, French and American, were thus hastened to the Myanmar coast as a sign of their governments' determination to prevent the supposed deaths of hundreds of thousands of innocent people.

It must be said that this time, unlike after the tsunami, the WHO posted on its website that corpses posed no risk and that survivors of the cyclone were in no danger of a deadly epidemic. But this was not enough to prevent the British Foreign Office from warning of the "peril", or to dissuade the advocates of armed interventionism, governments and associations alike, from using it to encourage the Security Council to activate the "Responsibility to protect" mechanism.[13]

Until the war in Libya in March 2011, instigated by the same governments (France, UK and the US), this was the only debate in which the Security Council had actually envisaged implementing this mechanism.

> Did emergency relief organisations learn any new lessons from the earthquake in Haiti?

The January 2010 earthquake in Haiti was the second mass medico-surgical emergency after the one in Pakistan in 2005. MSF had been working in Haiti for several years when the disaster struck and so was in the right place to respond rapidly. Three surgical units were set up in a container and the first major operations were performed three days after the earthquake. During the first forty-eight hours, care had been provided in the streets. The inflatable hospital used in Pakistan was sent out, so we were operating in optimum conditions from day thirteen, which is the time it took to get this really imposing piece of equipment on site and up and running. By the way, the famous forty-eight-hour window beyond which casualties cannot survive can now be filed away under "conventional wisdom", as the Pakistan precedent had already confirmed. MSF thus took up position alongside the multitude of local and international organisations, governmental and private, which had rushed to set up operations in Port-au-Prince and the surrounding region during the two weeks following the earthquake.

There was a lot of talk at the time about the chaos in which the "humanitarian expeditionary corps" was deployed. The lack of coordination and information on needs and the running of the relief operations were severely criticised in the press, but these criticisms don't actually hold water. Firstly, because disorder is the hallmark of a disaster, all the more so when it hits a country's capital and therefore its seat of power. Secondly, because the shortcomings of Haiti's public institutions were already notorious and the country was without an army, which had been dissolved under US pressure during the "Restore

Democracy" operation in 1995. Lastly (and most importantly), because the response to the urgent needs was focused on a limited area, it was carried out correctly, in spite of everything, with the notable exception of the shelters, which were both unsuitable and insufficient.

There are two medically-related issues that I would like to single out: the first, quite specific, concerns the use of techniques derived from war surgery, which tend to be more radical but can be inappropriate; the high number of military surgeons in such a setting, as well as the ever-present juxtapositions with the representation of war as mentioned earlier, give pause for thought. The other issue is more general and concerns the criteria adopted explicitly or otherwise by medical teams from different professional cultures[14] for deciding which cases, medical as well as surgical, should be given priority and which should not be treated. Do the exceptionally high workload and the logic of rationing induced by a disaster, which is where triage usually comes in, lead to laxity in procedures?[15] We have only fragmented and flimsy data, so I won't attempt to answer these questions. I just want to stress the need for a methodical reflection on them.

> Why is estimating the number of victims in a disaster the subject of such frequent debate?

Estimating the number of victims is another major issue as the figure is a crucial emotional marker, the trigger that "allows us to *feel* the disaster"[16] and determine where it features on the scale of gravity. Unlike what we see in many conflict situations, the disaster toll (usually an approximation) announced by the governmental authorities and the United Nations a few days after the event is accepted by the press and aid organisations as objective, in spite of its unreliability. Three days after the Haiti earthquake, the government announced that 50,000 bodies had been recovered. This figure was to increase day after day to reach 250,000, or even 300,000 a month later,[17] making the disaster one of the most serious ever.

These evaluations were based on an estimate of population density and the number of collapsed buildings in a given district, which left considerable room for uncertainty. Respect for the victims does not proscribe challenging figures drawn up in a chaotic environment and with no credible foundation. Heads of some of the UN agencies encountered six months after the earthquake privately agreed on a death toll of somewhere between 50,000 and 70,000, based mainly on the number of mass graves dug by Minustah, the only organisation charged with the task.[18] Similarly, after a survey of the different actors in their field, Handicap International Belgium's head of mission estimated that the number of disabled people was closer to 1,000 than 5,000, the figure that had ended up becoming official after being bandied about in aid circles.

Reducing the estimated loss of human life is clearly a sensitive issue, as it ties into collective emotion. Bringing down the numbers exposes us to suspicions of hard-heartedness, or even hostility or shameful ulterior motives, whether in situations of natural disaster or, even more so, in other settings with a more direct political dimension, such as armed conflict, population displacement, or the quantification of atrocities.[19] The death toll after the earthquake in Armenia in 1988, established at 100,000 deaths a few weeks after the disaster, was later reduced to 23,390 in figures published by the authorities. This reduction in the official death toll produced reactions of incomprehension, hostility even, as the original number had become a symbol of Armenian suffering and changing it was seen as a denial of this suffering. In practice, it is likely that such distortions and amplifications abound in many similar situations.

Estimating the number of victims—and the number of fatalities among them—is most definitely not a superfluous exercise, not only because this is the first question that everybody asks, but particularly because, however vague and fluctuating it may be while the aid is being set up, it allows a threshold effect to operate. It has been observed that we reason in terms of a major disaster justifying international-level deployment when the death toll reaches or exceeds ten thousand. The practical importance of such estimates from a relief agency's point of view is, however, limited, but I raise this issue here to underline how the highly uncertain nature of the figures makes it extremely difficult to know which resources to activate, other than basing ourselves on the threshold mentioned earlier. In concrete terms, the specific information required to guide relief operations would be, on the one hand, the number and condition of the survivors in order to gauge the medical assistance requirements, as well as needs for other types of aid—shelter, food, water, telecommunications, damage clearance and transport—and on the other, information on what the other relief operators, local as well as international, are doing.

234

Although not victims of an executioner, disaster victims are caught up in high stakes, as the examples given above have shown. Funding, media coverage, rallying sympathy for traumatised people, all combine to produce an escalation that nobody plans, but which is fostered by the apparently indisputable nature of the cause defended—that of increasing emergency aid as high as it can go.

Translated from French by Mandy Duret

IN THE NAME OF EMERGENCY
HOW MSF ADAPTS AND JUSTIFIES ITS CHOICES

Marc Le Pape

Given the constraints that MSF faces when it takes on, develops and supervises interventions, what justifications does it establish and choose to ensure that its actions are acceptable within its political, cultural, military and scientific environment and to those acting in its name?

The case studies in the first section of this book all take a dynamic approach to this question. This involves understanding processes and observing how MSF participates in them, defines its reasons for taking action and succeeds (or not) in implementing them. Each case presents the justifications for choosing and implementing programmes (including control, autonomy and speaking out) and recounts the local and international background that provide the context for these choices. The accounts illustrate justifications as they are being formed and, subsequently, as they are adapted based on the events that take place in each context and on the impacts of proposed programmes, medical practices and humanitarian arguments.

When conducting a sociological analysis of modes of justification, it is useful at the outset to identify characteristic attitudes that allow us

237

to make distinctions and identify ways of thinking. I will distinguish among realism, confrontation and abstention—three approaches and the three registers associated with them.

Realism, Confrontation and Abstention

An analysis of the cases described in this book illustrates the range of behaviours that the actors have adopted. I will initially address only those features that highlight differences and the heterogeneity of rationales for action in the face of actual or projected constraints. My approach draws on Albert Hirschman's characterisation of the three concepts of exit, voice and loyalty. I also rely on the sociological description of the realistic attitude, as presented by Cyril Lemieux.[1]

Hirschman's analysis addresses individual and collective responses to economic and political situations. He distinguishes among exit (that is, "simply leaving"), voice (the expression of discontent) and, last, loyalty, which involves the "intimation of some influence and the expectation that, over a period of time, the right turns will more than balance the wrong ones".[2] Hirschman seeks to identify the conditions in which these attitudes are expressed and the situations in which they contradict each other or work together.[3] According to Cyril Lemieux, the realistic attitude involves, for an individual and an organisation, recognising and accepting the limits of what can be done in a particular situation and drawing the appropriate conclusions; that is, exercising self-control, while attributing positive meaning to that cautious attitude.

I have chosen a "free"—as opposed to a literal—translation of Hirschman's three categories because this slight adaptation allows me to clarify several aspects of the choices made in MSF's areas of intervention. Thus, for "exit", I have chosen the term "abstention", for "voice", "confrontation" and, for "loyalty", "realism". These different terms do not mean that I have ignored Hirschman's lesson—quite the contrary. Indeed, he stated repeatedly that these concepts could be used to analyse a wide range of social phenomena and warned against applying them mechanically.

The terms chosen by the actors and observers to designate the logic behind certain choices may vary based on whether they attribute a positive or negative value to those choices. Thus, "realism" might be referred to as "collaboration" (with its negative meaning in France following World War II and the German occupation of the country) or "diplomacy". "Confrontation" could be seen as "irresponsibility" or "indignation". And last, "withdrawal" could be criticised as indifference or praised as a form of courage and professional rigour and as honouring MSF's principles. The perspective adopted is not intended to value or devalue, recommend one form of intervention over another or provide a guide to humanitarian arguments based on situations, moments in time, representatives or medical commitments. Rather, it represents a (partial) mapping of the range of choices and justifications actually adopted over the course of MSF's interventions during the decade 2000 to 2010, and does not suggest a preferred route.

There is a risk associated with this kind of description—that of creating "camps", as if the proponents of each way of thinking form a camp, as if "caught by compelling reflexes and lumbering predictably through set motions and manoeuvres".[4] We will see that MSF is not home to camps that assert a particular way of thinking but, rather, that those who adopt the realistic position in a given situation will, at another point in the process, endorse confrontation or abstention, and vice-versa.

I will now describe how these attitudes are expressed in MSF's projects.

Which Practices are Associated with Realism?

The general feature of the "realistic" attitude is the unchallenged acceptance of constraints imposed by national and international authorities in order to preserve opportunities for action. This involves conciliation, either in the interest of obtaining authorisation to initiate and, subsequently, develop an activity or to preserve the possibility of future action.

MSF-Holland's intervention in Myanmar, which began in 1992, typifies this choice. To establish a presence there, the organisation initially relinquished its project to intervene in Rakhine State, where the government was brutally repressing the Rohingya minority, and accepted the site on the outskirts of Yangon that the government assigned it. The Swiss section made the same kind of concession in exchange for permission to enter the country in 1999. The second category of concessions dealt with control over the programme. Starting in late 2004, the government imposed more complicated procedures for entering the country, tightened the rules for travelling outside of Yangon, demanded that aid organisations submit lists of their employees, and required that a "liaison officer" accompany teams in their travels. In short, the government increased the restrictions limiting the autonomy of the medical teams. The third category of concessions involved the agreement made by the two MSF sections was not to publicly criticise the authorities, including criticism of the restrictions placed on their medical activities.

In order to treat malnutrition in India, MSF's Spanish section chose to limit the visibility of its activities, restrict its work to a single district and focus on treating severe acute malnutrition. However, MSF's nutritional programmes involve importing ready-to-use therapeutic foods (RUTF), which activists from the Right to Food campaign (with whom MSF was in discussions) criticised and the national government disapproved of. However, thanks to the limitations it had placed on its activities, MSF-Spain succeeded in signing a district-level agreement. The medical authorities then agreed to allow the organisation to use RUTF to treat severe acute malnutrition.

Facing obstacles at the local level, MSF-France chose to abandon its project and withdraw quietly. This form of withdrawal characterises both the confrontational attitude—expressed by a refusal to continue negotiating—and the realistic attitude, as demonstrated by the discretion with which it withdrew. Because the withdrawal was limited to one project, MSF was able to continue to participate in debates within India over the treatment of malnutrition.

Indeed, each case study reveals moments when the realistic attitude comes into play. Constraints exist everywhere and differ only in their intensity, reach and nature. We must learn to live with them and negotiate ways of adapting our actions to comply with them. Each situation raises the question of acceptable limits. The realistic phase of the action allows us to learn lessons from which we can assess the extent to which the humanitarian work is compatible with the constraints and, then to decide whether to continue, confront or withdraw. That is why it is useful to present situations that highlight the choice to adopt the realistic approach, as in the case studies dealing with Sri Lanka, Nigeria, the Gaza Strip, Somalia, Afghanistan and Yemen.

What Does Confrontation Mean Within MSF?

Negotiation is a form of confrontation, but it is, at first, a discreet and contained form as its goal is to reach agreements, in the spirit of realism, since MSF seeks to be able to carry out medical activities. This was the case in Afghanistan when, in 2008, MSF sought to resume the activities it had halted in 2004 after five of its members were killed. In 2008 to 2009, negotiations were undertaken on several fronts, including with US authorities. To ensure the safety of patients (whether affiliated with the opposition or not) in Lashkar Gah hospital where MSF was working, the facility had to be designated as neutral and the presence of armed men thus prohibited under the Geneva Conventions. The goal of negotiations with the armed opponents of the Karzai government was to reach an agreement allowing drugs to be transported safely on the roads. Confrontation with the US authorities was avoided when the Obama administration issued directives to the US military command that satisfied the demands MSF had made locally. However, confrontation with the armed opponents proved difficult to contain through negotiation. The representatives of the Islamic Emirate of Afghanistan (IEA) took advantage of MSF's requests to make demands that were difficult for the latter to meet—for example, a signed commitment from the US military forces guaranteeing their compliance with the Geneva Conventions, which MSF was not in a position to obtain. Using its ability to permit or block the transport of drugs, the IEA initiated a confrontation that MSF was forced to take up and through which the government's opponents sought political gain; that is, recognition and legitimisation of their power in the areas they controlled.

However, the tensions did not confine themselves to discreet discussions with the various parties holding power and men of influence, from the local level to that of States and international institutions. The organisation's policy in South Africa is characteristic of entering the realm of public confrontation. Allied with the Treatment Action Campaign (TAC), an activist movement that organises HIV/AIDS treatment, MSF supported TAC in its campaign against authorities whose public positions were clearly influenced by theories denying that a virus causes the illness. The campaign specifically targeted the minister of health and President Thabo Mbeki, whose position led the government to refuse to provide antiretroviral treatment to patients. Between 2008 and 2010, MSF worked with legal organisations, this time to defend the rights of Zimbabwean immigrants in South Africa to obtain medical care. In early 2008, MSF had launched medical aid programmes targeting that population along the border with Zimbabwe and in Johannesburg. It used the information gathered during medical consultations and provided its expertise to strengthen the activists' efforts to obtain access to healthcare for immigrants.

The organisation has been involved in other forms of public critique, for example, in Ethiopia, where MSF-Switzerland closed its mission and simultaneously issued a press release denouncing the obstacles imposed by authorities on its medical activities in the Somali region. "Despite continuous attempts to improve the working relations with the authorities, our organisation can only regret the absence of any space to bring independent and impartial assistance".[5] In another example, MSF-France participated in several public campaigns supporting universal healthcare coverage and, subsequently, working with other organisations, advocated for the continued right of foreigners who are ill "to remain in France legally and continue to receive medical treatment".[6] In the former example, the organisation asked the Ethiopian government to allow it to take action and in the latter, it encouraged the French government to take action.

The strategy of roundly criticising institutions, as in the South African case and many other situations,[7] is far from the most common approach. In fact, MSF usually prefers to confine confrontation to the negotiating process. This reality contrasts with the general image of the organisation—a powerful media presence, effective in its use of public criticism and capable of harming businesses, governments and international bodies through its interventions.

Abstention

MSF adopts this behaviour regularly as establishing medical priorities means choosing certain interventions and, simultaneously, rejecting others. Marie-Pierre Allié, president of the French section, has thus stated "It is our duty to find solutions for the patients whom we have started to treat, but that does not commit us to providing care to the entire population in a given location forever".[8] However, the boundaries between intervention and abstention are becoming increasingly unclear in MSF's work. Whereas MSF has long chosen not to address chronic infections requiring long-term treatment, the organisation currently treats patients suffering from tuberculosis and AIDS, which require treatment that may last for several months (the former) or a lifetime (the latter).

The decision to abstain or intervene provokes debates that reach beyond medical issues. Both choices have generated and regularly generate controversies, even confrontations, among MSF actors. Some support the termination of a programme on the basis that MSF is an emergency response group, shifting the discussion from the medical register to the political register, and transforming controversy into confrontation. Such an attempt to confine MSF to a narrow identity would be in mere contradiction with its actual practices, all the more observing the adaptability of the principles guiding its actions and the range of situations in which it intervenes. The identity-based argument continues to exercise a certain influence within MSF, but it is effective only if supported by those with the power to make decisions and control communications within the national sections of the organisation. This characterises the situation in which MSF-France chose to leave northern Nigeria quietly. In 2005, it opened a programme to treat severe acute malnutrition in Katsina State. When *Reuters* news agency reported on the nutritional crisis in the region,[9] the minister of health, fearing the negative image conveyed by crowds of emaciated children, pushed to close the programme. MSF-France threatened to make a public statement, but when it observed the declining number of children in need of treatment, it abandoned the threat and quietly left Katsina in December 2005. During the same period, and in the years that followed, the same section adopted an entirely different approach to malnutrition in Niger, one characterised by both realism and confrontation, "transforming limitations into challenges and challenges into choices".[10]

The Basis of the Justifications

To characterise more accurately the arguments supporting one approach over another—specifically, realism over confrontation (or the contrary)—we must place these choices in the context of missions, as recounted by the authors of the case studies.

Realism

As we have seen, realism appears first as a necessity. Agreement must be reached with the "powers that be". These negotiations are thus part of the typical work of MSF staff in order to open, set up, maintain and develop a mission. We are not focused here on the moment at which the realism critical to the start of a mission comes into play, but rather on how this attitude is maintained, even when the circumstances might lead to confrontation in its most diverse forms. The dominant argument asserted most regularly to justify realism is the threat of danger. It is commonly linked with the argument that criticism is pointless and "cannot make any real difference".[11]

Several threats are raised, often simultaneously, as in 2009, when the MSF-France head of mission in Sri Lanka made the case for cautious silence. "What should our communications strategy be when we do not have first-hand information to convey? When an organisation present in the conflict zone (i.e., the ICRC)—and thus with greater legitimacy in discussing the situation—already has an international communications structure in place? When it is fairly clear that it will have no effect on the people on whose behalf we want to intervene? When, from an operational perspective, MSF lacked the ability to respond that would have allowed us to really confront the authorities? When it has a significant risk of exposing the national staff?"[12]

Realism is justified primarily by three dangers: that of abandoning patients and halting treatments; of endangering the field teams' national staff members;[13] and of being prohibited from expanding the area of intervention, risking expulsion and undermining future opportunities to intervene.

The Sri Lanka missions provide examples of the decision not to issue public criticism in the name of medical emergency. In 2009, the Sri Lankan army broke through the defence lines of the rebel Tamil Tigers, who controlled an increasingly limited amount of territory. Tens of thousands of civilians were evacuated from rebel zones to a transit area and then forced to gather in internment camps, referred to officially as "welfare villages". MSF-France was initially involved near the Menik Farm camp, where it set up a surgical hospital. The programme was covered under an agreement with the Ministry of Health, but the agreement came at a price—a confidentiality clause under which MSF would refrain from any "public comment" without the approval of the Ministry of Health. This was a severe constraint for MSF, but the organisation accepted it in order to avoid expulsion, and with the goal of reducing restrictions on access to the camps so that it could provide medical assistance to internees. The restrictions remained in place. The medical work to be carried out and the proposal to expand the intervention in the camps justified that perseverance, at least in the eyes of those supporting that choice. An evaluation drafted after several MSF managers visited Sri Lanka expresses that view. "There is no shortage of work to be done on 'the Farm' [the Menik Farm camp]. We should become a vital cog in its operations, because that's the only way we'll have a chance to eliminate it (or make a stir getting out) when we think the time is right".[14]

The desire to respond to the population's "medical needs" and not to abandon "our patients" at any price was the overwhelming motive for staying in Myanmar. An MSF-Holland programme manager stated that clearly in 2007 on *CNN*. "We have a very large programme. Last year, we treated more than a million patients for malaria and AIDS. The programme activities are still going on. We are treating deadly diseases. So it is very important for us to continue the treatment of the patients". This choice justified avoiding actions that could put the medical activities at risk, regardless of what was happening in Myanmar. The field coordinators also feared that any criticism of the regime could lead to reprisals against the organisation's Burmese employees and endanger them. The teams working in Sri Lanka expressed the same fear. In fact, the dangers facing teams suggest that such fears are quite legitimate. In the Ogaden region of Ethiopia, national staff members were accused of spying and some were jailed. In Palestine, two Gazan employees were questioned harshly by Hamas police officers and, on 4 August 2006, seventeen employees of Action Contre la Faim were executed in Sri Lanka.

We have already noted the justification for choosing not to issue public criticism because it would make no difference—not in general, but in specific cases such as in Sri Lanka, when the MSF-France head of mission concluded that public comment "will have no effect on the people on whose behalf we want to intervene". The futility of issuing condemnations was also put forth after the September 2009 bombing of civilians in Al Talh, Yemen. The government air force carried out the attack, which MSF-France witnessed. It was the only aid organisation present and also treated several seriously injured children at the hospital, only two of whom survived. However, the organisation chose not to condemn the bombing, concluding that such an action would not lead the belligerents to adopt less fierce methods of combat, but could threaten MSF's medical activities and disrupt its relationship with the Yemeni government, which was critical to MSF's ability to carry out its work. That relationship had to be preserved as humanitarian aid could not be deployed without it.

The futility argument has been asserted under other circumstances. In 2001, the MSF team in the Gaza Strip challenged the Paris operational centre, criticising it for ignoring the experience in the field and the statements the team had gathered to condemn Israel's treatment of the Palestinian people. Several MSF-France board members responded that the Palestinian situation is one of the world's leading news stories and that the statements gathered by MSF dealt with violence that had already received extensive coverage. The term "futile" was not used explicitly as it would have shocked its audience. However, that was the political subtext of the critique of using the statements to express an emotional and political commitment to a population subjected, here, to constant violence from operations conducted by the Israeli army.

Confrontation

The choice to confront is based on several justifications: first, "imminent danger", according to which "it is not good enough to argue for a certain policy on the ground that it is *right;* one must urge that it is imperatively needed to stave off some threatening disaster";[15] second, respect for international humanitarian law; and, third, agreement with the principles set forth in the MSF charter and several "reference documents" in which the organisation sets forth its rules for intervening and reasons for taking action.

The 2005 nutritional crisis in Niger offers a representative example of how the imminent danger argument is used. In April, MSF-France observed and publicly stated that an unusually high number of children were suffering from severe acute malnutrition and called for "general food distributions". In early June the demand became more pressing. "Exceptional measures must be undertaken urgently so that the most vulnerable populations can gain direct, free access to food". In late June another public statement was issued. It described the imminent danger in sharper terms than prior communications. "There will be thousands of avoidable deaths this summer", it stated, referring to children who would die, despite the existence of nutritional products that could save them.[16] MSF regularly issues announcements of life-threatening risks. In general, they seek to alert national and international authorities and trigger action on their part. They correspond to a standard medical position. First, a diagnosis and a corresponding prescription exist. Second, MSF's experts and epidemiologists have assessed the efficacy of these prescriptions in their practice and their surveys. A standard medical demand thus follows, justifying public confrontation when the organisation believes that institutions are resisting treatments with proven therapeutic affect. MSF has often undertaken this kind of confrontation to obtain acceptance of a new treatment; for example, to justify the introduction and prescription of antiretrovirals and tritherapies for HIV, and of artemesin-derived combination drug therapies in malaria epidemics when resistance to the anti-malarials previously used in Africa was recognised.[17] Some link these initiatives and the political work they involve to the "universal medical ethics" referred to in the MSF charter, while others summon a professional code of ethics. Regardless, a public statement identifying a neglected danger inevitably transforms the doctor's report into a political critique. The authorities it criticises will certainly respond—either by prohibiting certain activities, imposing additional bureaucratic obstacles, expelling the organisation or threatening to do so.

International humanitarian law[18] is evoked regularly when the organisation's unfettered access to populations it believes require aid is blocked. This was the case in Sri Lanka, Ogaden and Pakistan. Other references to standards are also raised, particularly those developed in the set of texts in which MSF defines the principles of medical-humanitarian action it respects; specifically, impartiality in providing care, the prohibition against weapons at sites where medical care is provided and "complete independence from all governments and political, economic and religious powers" (the MSF charter). When these principles are evoked in a public setting to support an argument, they are presented as lines that the organisation may not cross. However, even when it comes to these principles, advocates of realism can undermine advocates of confrontation. Concessions may thus be made in terms of the rules presented as essential to medical humanitarian action, such as the personal participation of MSF staff in providing medical care, the final choice of medical priorities to which MSF commits and programmes being overseen by MSF's doctors.

Abstention

The argument regularly asserted in support of abstention can be summarised as follows: "That's not MSF's role". There are several versions of that argument. One refers to MSF's "identity" and the other relies on the language of the medical practitioner, emphasising MSF's expertise and medical priorities to reject certain activities. In the latter case, abstention comes into play in the case of medical controversies that could become internal political confrontations when the issue of identity is advanced to impose or condemn a decision.

The case studies do not include many examples of such confrontations. Rather, the writers focus on accounts of what the MSF sections wanted to do and, subsequently, were able to do. They rarely refer to diseases that the sections chose not to treat. To understand the choice to abstain would require new investigations, specifically regarding the debates that arise when programmes are defined.

Between Realism and Confrontation: Inevitable Tensions and Interactions

Does the register of realism prevail in situations characterised by armed conflict and confrontation in peaceful ones? Indeed, in the absence of armed conflicts, there is a more systematic reliance on public criticism, confrontation and alliances with other organisations, as can be seen in the cases of South Africa and France. However, in practice, if we observe missions from start to finish, they are rarely characterised by a single style. Rather, there is almost always a shift from one kind of reasoning and register to another. This works both ways—from realism to confrontation and from confrontation to realism. These variations are related to the dynamics of each situation.

Nonetheless, the different forms of reasoning the organisation relies on may be contradictory, provoking conflicts and even crises inside the movement[19] and its sections. Thus, those who opt for confrontation and public criticism value the approach when it produces a change that some consider progress in medical practice. However, it is questioned by others who emphasise obstacles blocking current programmes and obstructing their development. Those who advocate and practise the realistic approach in certain situations view it positively, as they believe it allows medical programmes to be implemented, even in extremely restrictive contexts. Those who take a negative viewpoint consider the concessions unacceptable in the name of the principles of humanitarian action and medical goals that they believe define MSF. Last, those who support abstention rely on the fact that certain illnesses require long-term treatment that they consider to be incompatible with MSF's actions and responsibilities. Their critics condemn abstention and withdrawal as a form of irresponsibility toward patients—a refusal to commit on a long-term basis and a sign of the conservative nature of MSF's medical practices.

The fact that we observe changes in the way certain approaches are valued and that the way they are described shifts from positive to negative and back again does not mean that we cannot resolve uncertainty surrounding the validity of choices. However, we must not always stand with the universal—"to claim supposedly universal principles" such as the Geneva Conventions—but must reach a compromise between the universal and the specific, invoking this particular actor's unique medical experience to justify critiques of governmental measures or, conversely, the need to accommodate them. Indeed, "these two modes of legitimisation are not mutually exclusive. In most cases, one may even find that they are both required in order to lodge a complaint or justify an action".[20]

In 2006, the MSF movement collectively reaffirmed several action principles. First among them, "the individual medical-humanitarian act [...] is central to the work of MSF".[21] This principle exists in contrast with another "essential role", that of publicly condemning "grave and ignored crimes" and "massive and neglected acts of violence against individuals and groups"[22] that actors in the field can witness based on medical data and their own experience.

We have seen that the tension between medical action and speaking out is, in fact, inherent to the organisation's work and may always provoke contradictory judgments that are, to a lesser or greater degree, inflexible. This is what I sought to reconstruct by presenting the many justifications that MSF's actors rely on to make medical programmes acceptable or, in other words, to be compatible with the many constraints facing doctors in humanitarian settings before they can take action, while medical programmes are being developed and, finally, when it is time to end those programmes. I have tried not to take sides. Some may certainly challenge that stance, particularly those who take action must make, justify and defend their choices—and accept the consequences. Nonetheless, placing myself at a distance (but not on a higher plane) is useful if it allows me to reconstruct the many ways of responding to constraints on action that MSF has adopted over the course of the 2000s.

AFTERWORD

David Rieff

There was never any room for compromise in the myth of the "French doctors". Aid was a moral imperative, full stop. Like all doctrines founded on such an absolute (not to say absolutely self-righteous) conception, moral ambiguity was taboo, and the need for negotiation seen as, at best, a necessary evil. To be sure, most international relief groups, and certainly MSF, have moved beyond this kind of vulgar Kantianism which Bernard Kouchner once championed so insistently. Nonetheless, in the collective memory of modern humanitarianism, the comforting illusion endures that there was a time when relief NGOs were largely free to act as they saw fit, taking into account only the needs of the populations they sought to help, and the limits imposed by their own charters. Populations in danger, to use an expression that MSF made into a commonplace of the humanitarian lexicon more than a decade ago, were assumed to have the right to be helped but, just as saliently, international relief groups took it as read that they had an absolute right to help. In reality, humanitarian action cannot afford to be absolutist in, say, the manner of the human rights movement, which, because it is law based, is absolutist, at least in principle, or it is nothing. All effective humanitarian action is based on negotiating compromises with the relevant political actors, including of course insurgent groups, donors, and with other stakeholders (including beneficiaries, themselves never monolithic in their view-points or requirements), and trying to reconcile competing agendas,

251

not only between NGOs but within NGOs as well. For a humanitarian organisation to believe and, far more importantly, to behave as if this were not the case is to court disaster, as a number of the case studies in this book painfully illustrate.

The need for compromise in almost every situation in which an organisation like MSF operates or is likely to operate emphatically does not imply that, where the compromises on offer are unacceptable from a relief NGO's perspective, it is imperative to act anyway. That would not be compromise, but rather a supine capitulation. Instead, as Fiona Terry puts it in her chapter on Myanmar, what is essential is for there to be an emphasis on internal discussions "of [the] parameters or benchmarks against which to judge acceptable from unacceptable compromises". The French title of this book is *Agir à tout prix?* (*Acting at any price?*). It is posed as a question, but in fact it is only a rhetorical one, since MSF's answer to it is an emphatic "No". It is difficult to see how any other answer could be acceptable. There are times where it may appear to an outsider that MSF as an institution wished that it could make such a claim, but the legal mandate that provides the moral, as well as the operational, rationale for the International Committee of the Red Cross' practice of operating everywhere that security constraints do not preclude it from doing so without subjecting its delegates to intolerable risk is simply unavailable to the association. But following in the footsteps of the caritative arms of the United Nations system and never withdrawing whatever the negative effects of their relief efforts may be (the genocidaire controlled Hutu refugee camps in eastern Zaire in the aftermath of the Rwandan genocide are the emblematic example of this) is available, but is rightly viewed as being unacceptable. Faced with such a dilemma, MSF has little choice but to jealously guard what Rony Brauman has called its "right of abstention", for given the fact that compromise is a far greater imperative in humanitarian action than the "*droit d'ingérence*", not acting at any price and in all circumstances, no matter how unfavourable, becomes the sine qua non for an international aid organisation to maintain its autonomy.

That is why, however paradoxical it may appear to be at first glance, the connection between compromise and autonomy actually is a central one. It is true that impartiality and neutrality have figured more prominently in the collective imagination of the humanitarian international (and nowhere more so than within MSF), but if there has been one idea that has been invaluable in practice, at the practical level, it has been autonomy. This should not be surprising. Neutrality and impartiality are important as ideas, but they beg as many questions as they illuminate, and even when understood as contingent rather than unvarying concepts, leave much to be desired. Impartiality in humanitarian action is one of those concepts that, like objectivity in journalism, is a goal rather than a reality, rather like the horizon in ocean navigation before the advent of GPS. As for neutrality, well, the political contradictions and moral and ethical limitations of that idea are both too obvious and too well rehearsed to need much further elaboration. In contrast, as an American Supreme Court judge once famously said of pornography, we all know autonomy when we see it. It is commonplace for moral philosophers to identify the so-called objective correlatives of a given word or idea. But these are far easier to grasp when the subject is humanitarian autonomy than they are when it is impartiality or neutrality that are being discussed.

Caveat lector: One cannot speak about absolute autonomy here. That is no more an attainable goal for MSF, or any other humanitarian association, than absolute anything else. But whatever else has changed in the four decades since MSF's founding, experience has shown that often always and in all circumstances, a reasonable degree of autonomy can be obtained and maintained provided that a particular action or programme is coherent in its understanding of the conditions in which the association will work (above all in the sense of the limitations that governments and insurgent groups are likely to put on these efforts); realistic in its acknowledgment of the ever shifting and inevitably contingent nature of the conditions on the ground that must determine whether a humanitarian relief organisation continues to operate; or if the crossing of too many deontological red lines forces the group to give serious thought to withdrawing—caveats that apply to all the understandings made by the NGO with local actors as well. As every practitioner knows, these are treacherous waters in which to swim. The solution certainly does not lie in securing enough humanitarian space (a parlous concept in any case, and one that whatever its past utility should be definitively retired for any number of reasons, including those Marie-Pierre Allié adduces in her introduction to this book), let alone of falling for the fantasy that humanitarian action can ever exist in some sort of splendid isolation from the contexts in which it is undertaken. The relevance of the idea of autonomy derives from its essentially transactional nature—at least when applied to the humanitarian context. One does not simply assert one's autonomy, one defends it. In contrast, humanitarian space is a sentimental idea, neutrality a bogus one, and impartiality an abstraction, however necessary, and it is a lost cause to try to defend any of them. The sooner they are given a decent burial, the sooner we can all move on.

If the answer to one of the key questions posed by this book in a number of different ways, sometimes explicit, sometimes implicit, is that there can be no true autonomy for humanitarian actors without the right of abstention, the ghost at the banquet is whether maintaining even a tenuous autonomy for humanitarian action is still a realistic possibility in the battle spaces of the so-called Long War (or Global War on Terrorism, or whatever it is being called this week), from Afghanistan and Pakistan, through the Yemen to the Horn, and then on to the Sahelian countries. Xavier Crombé and Michiel Hofman's essay on MSF in Afghanistan and Jonathan Whittall's essay on the association's work in Pakistan in this book answer with a qualified yes. They acknowledge that in both places there have been systematic efforts to enlist humanitarian relief efforts in the service of winning the hearts and minds of the population. To be sure, humanitarian action in one form or another has frequently been an integral part of counter-insurgency strategy going back to the British in Malaya.[1] What is different in Afghanistan and Pakistan has been the centrality of humanitarian action in the broadest sense of the term. To paraphrase Clausewitz, humanitarianism, not just war, has now become the continuation of politics by other means. Nonetheless, Crombé, Hofman, and Whittall argue strongly that MSF has had some success in resisting these attempts at co-optation by US-led ISAF forces in Afghanistan, and the government in Islamabad and the US Agency for International Development in Pakistan, and, instead, convincing both the government and the insurgent side that MSF's medical assistance could be useful enough to both to be allowed to continue, at least for the time being. In the Pakistani case, MSF's ability to draw a distinction between its own conception of humanitarian assistance and those of most other mainline NGOs, pursuing programmes more in sync with the regime's (and Washington's) counter-insurgency goals, has led to a measure of acceptance by the insurgency.

How long this can continue is an open question. There are already laws on the books in the United States that criminalise any aid provided to terrorist groups. On some readings of this law, setting up a hospital, or even providing support for a medical programme in an area controlled by the Taliban or similar groups could leave MSF open to prosecution for "supporting" terrorism. But even assuming, as seems most likely at the present moment at least, that no such charges are ever brought, it is not clear that Washington would tolerate a significant expansion of MSF or any other relief NGO's efforts in Taliban controlled areas. After all, if success in counter-insurgency is more contingent on winning hearts and minds than on killing the enemy (and today, the near universal consensus is that it is), then aid distributed in insurgent areas with the accord of the guerrillas will presumably have the opposite effect. Were that effect to start to be seen in Kabul or Islamabad as significant, it seems doubtful that it would be allowed to continue without sanction as it has been so far. For the moment, however, the fact that MSF can negotiate with all sides, and secure their assent if not their approval to act with some autonomy in government and insurgent dominated areas alike—thus separating itself to what to an outsider seems like a remarkable degree from the humanitarianism in the service of the state that is the reigning ethos of the battle space— is a testimony to the transactional basis of humanitarian autonomy in the present moment.

Because MSF mostly relies on private funds, it has been better able to resist being "integrated" into so-called post-conflict reconstruction efforts than most of the other important mainline relief NGOs. Nonetheless, if the MSF position on these matters has a weakness, it is in the association's confidence, which at times well and truly crosses the line and tumbles over into vanity, that it can somehow stand apart from the humanitarian system—and, like it or not, there is only that one system, for all the important divergences and ethical standpoints between the actors within it—whilst simultaneously participating in it. Surely, legitimate questions can be asked about both the operational and the moral and political significance of a right of abstention if, in exercising it, MSF does so in the full knowledge that another organisation will rush in to carry out the role it declined to play, or decided no longer to fulfill. It was this perception that lay at the heart of the criticism, notably by Sergio Vieira de Mello when he was still assistant high commissioner of UNHCR, of MSF's decision to withdraw from the refugee camps of eastern Zaire. In his article on Sri Lanka, Fabrice Weissman bravely acknowledges the extent to which MSF has fallen victim to its own tendency to think of itself as an "NGO apart". "Having returned to Sri Lanka thinking itself the beneficiary of a special status in the world of international solidarity", he writes, "MSF found itself in an extremely fragile negotiating position, which in the end was comparable to that of other NGOs". Trying to predict the future is rarely a very useful exercise, but it seems entirely safe to predict that the dilemmas it faced in the last period of the war in Sri Lanka and in the immediate aftermath of the crushing of the Tamil LTTE insurgency will confront it time and again in the years to come, and that this is not the last time it will feel obliged to bow to the "diktats", to use Weissman's terms, of the government of a country in which it is trying to work.

The consequences of this are considerable. Not only should MSF and groups choosing to follow its "independentist" (as opposed to "statist") humanitarian line not delude themselves that the only question that needs to be asked is "Faut-il agir à tout prix?", they should also leave the mental space for what they all know to be the essentially tragic nature of their action—once described by Philippe Gaillard of the ICRC as "injecting a measure of humanity, always insufficient, into situations that should not exist". MSF-France, with its history of scepticism (never fully shared by the other sections of the association, let alone by other mainline relief NGOs, and now unfortunately weakened even in Paris...) about all grandiose claims, whether in the mould of a Kouchner or of Oxfam, for what humanitarian action can accomplish, should be particularly alert to the limitations of their own agency. While the authors of this book are absolutely correct when they insist that, as Marie-Pierre Allié puts it, rather than speaking of a defined and immutable humanitarian space (shrinking or otherwise), it is more truthful to speak of humanitarian actors having a "space for negotiations [in the context of the] relations of force and of interest between aid groups and the authorities", it is not mere declinism to ask whether those relations of force are likely to grow ever more unfavourable to MSF and like-minded organisations. Speaking of MSF's initial attempts to resist playing the role that the Ethiopian government wanted to assign it in Ogaden, Laurence Binet, in her contribution to the book, writes sardonically of MSF having "resisted the first waltz", but in the end having "bent to the tempo that permitted it to stay at the dance".

These examples—and, to Sri Lanka and Ethiopia, one could reasonably add the Sudanese government's behaviour toward the humanitarian NGOs in Darfur—should make it clear that while the limitations put on humanitarian autonomy by the political and military goals of the global war on terrorism are real enough, they are scarcely the only challenge faced by humanitarian actors in the second decade of the twenty-first century. Indeed, if the contributors to this book are correct, then MSF has been more successful in securing a measure of autonomy for itself from the Americans, the Pakistanis, and the Taliban, than they have from strong states in the Global South where the conflicts that are occurring have little or nothing to do with Jihadism. Of course, this may not last, but if it doesn't that will not be because the authorities in Colombo, Addis Ababa, and Khartoum, following a trend that began in Rwanda after the Rwandan Patriotic Front took power in 1994, have grown less exigent, but rather because ISAF or the Quetta Shura have grown more so. But the increasingly unfavourable relations of force between these governments and MSF can be seen in the association's developing reluctance to make public statements—above all, those that involved generalising about the humanitarian situation, a demarche whose repercussions, once it has been undertaken are usually very difficult to control—lest it provoke retaliation from the regimes concerned. These concerns were entirely warranted, as is evidenced by MSF's experience of having been expelled from Darfur and Niger, and threatened with expulsion from Sri Lanka, Ethiopia, and Yemen (in this last case not least for having dared to put Yemen on the list of what, in any case, was MSF's extremely ill-judged annual "Top Ten Humanitarian Crises" media campaign).[2] And they bode ill for the future, since there is every reason for other states wishing to bring humanitarian groups to heel, and having observed how effective such measures are, from taking similar steps.

Having said all that, the situation is scarcely hopeless. As several contributors to this book point out, there are very few governments or insurgent groups (even among the most militant Jihadis) who challenge the basic premise of international humanitarian aid or challenge its claim to at least some degree of political autonomy. Instead, as the Afghan case illustrates, the debate is over whether relief groups are, in fact, taking sides. The insistence of US government officials, from Colin Powell and Andrew Natsios during the Bush administration to Hillary Clinton and Samantha Power under Barack Obama, that relief NGOs not try to distance themselves but rather develop closer links to US and other ISAF forces has done a great deal of harm to the efforts of MSF and other humanitarian organisations seeking to work wherever the needs were most urgent, rather than where they would do the most good for the Coalition's war effort. Nevertheless, MSF has succeeded to a remarkable extent in distancing itself from that project with the result that it has been able to operate in at least some Taliban areas. Surely the same approach can bear fruit in the future in other theatres of war. Is this enough? Self-evidently, it is anything but enough. But in a time when fanatics on all sides seem willing to accept nothing less than the total defeat and unconditional surrender of their foes, it may be as much as we have any right to expect. Sometimes just holding the line for one's values as best one can, making the compromises that one must, and playing the long game in the full knowledge that relations of force are always changing, and not always for the worse, is no small victory.

NOTES

INTRODUCTION

1. MSF is an international movement with nineteen sections, overseen by boards of directors, and grouped into five operational platforms in France, Belgium, Holland, Switzerland and Spain.
2. Echo, "The humanitarian space under pressure", http://ec.europa.eu.
3. "L'espace humanitaire en danger", Université d'automne de l'humanitaire, 4th édition. 28–30 Sept. 2006: proceedings.
4. Quoted in "Humanitarian action under siege", OCHA, 18 Aug. 2009.
5. Don Hubert, Cynthia Brassard Boudreau, "Shrinking humanitarian space? Trends and prospects on security and access", *The Journal of Humanitarian Assistance*, 24 Nov. 2010.
6. Fabrice Weissman (ed.), *In the Shadow of Just Wars: Violence, Politics and Humanitarian Action*, London: Hurst & Co. Publishers Ltd, 2004.
7. MSF's first charter, 1971.
8. Rony Brauman, president's report, 1987, MSF-France.
9. See after, Fabrice Weissman, "Silence heals...", pp. 177–97.
10. Paul Ricœur, "Foreword", Medical commission of Amnesty International's French section, and Valérie Marange, *Médecins tortionnaires, médecins résistants*, Paris: La Découverte, 1989.
11. Paul Ricœur, "Pour une éthique du compromis". Interviews by Jean-Marie Muller and François Vaillant, *Alternatives non violentes*, n° 80, Oct. 1991.
12. Ricoeur, "Pour une éthique du compromis".
13. See after, Jean-Hervé Bradol, "Caring for health", p. 216.
14. Jean-Hervé Bradol, "Introduction", Fabrice Weissman (ed.), *In the Shadow of Just Wars...*, p. 9.
15. See after, Jean-Hervé Bradol, "Caring for health", op. cit.
16. Michel Feher, "Les gouvernés en politique", *Vacarme*, n° 34, Winter 2006.
17. See after, Marc Le Pape, "In the name of emergency", p. 242.

PART ONE: STORIES

1. SRI LANKA: AMID ALL-OUT WAR

1. Cf. for example, V.K. Shashikumar, "Lessons from the War in Sri Lanka", *Indian Defence Review*, 24, no. 3 (July–Sept. 2009); Lawrence Hart, "The option no one wants to think about", *The Jerusalem Post*, 9 Dec. 2009.

2. Eric Meyer and Eleanor Pavey, "Bons offices, surveillance, médiation: les ratés du processus de paix à Sri Lanka" [Good offices, surveillance and mediation: failures in the Sri Lankan peace process], in *Critique Internationale*, no. 22 Jan. 2004, 35–46, p. 37.

3. Jayadeva Uyangoda, "The Way We Are. Politics of Sri Lanka 2007–2008", Colombo: Social Scientists' Association, 2008, p. 7.

4. Report of the Secretary-General's Panel of Experts on Accountability in Sri Lanka, United Nations, 31 Mar. 2011.

5. Cf., for example, "Offensive to provide water, not to gain territory", *The Sunday Leader*, Volume 13, Issue 4 Colombo, 6 Aug. 2006.

6. Ministry of Defence—Sri Lanka, "Ultimatum to LTTE expires: terrorists ignore safe passage for stranded civilians", 1 Feb. 2009, http://www.defence.lk/new.asp?fname=20090201_01.

7. Report of the Secretary General's Panel of Experts on Accountability in Sri Lanka, UN.

8. ICG, "War Crimes in Sri Lanka', Brussels: International Crisis Group", 17 May 2010.

9. UTHR(J), *Can the East be Won Through Human Culling?*, Special Report no. 26, University Teachers for Human Rights (Jaffna), Aug. 2007, http://www.uthr.org/SpecialReports/spreport26.hhhtm.

10. Cf., on this topic, Simon Harris, "Humanitarianism in Sri Lanka: Lessons Learned", Feinstein International Center, Tufts University, Briefing Paper, June 2010, https://wikis.uit.tufts.edu/confluence/pages/viewpage.action?pageId=36675391.

11. MSF-Holland, Sri Lanka Annual Plans 2008 and 2009.

12. Interview with the former MSF-France head of mission on 24 Feb. 2011.

13. Cf., for example "Four INGOs to be booted out over link with Tigers", *The Island*, 30 Sept. 2006; "Ignominious departure for INGOs, under fire for alleged assistance to LTTE and non-implementation of post-tsunami rebuilding pledges", *The Sunday Times*, 8 Oct. 2006.

14. Jeremy Page, "Barbed wire villages raise fears of refugee concentration camps", *The Times*, 13 Feb. 2009.

15. Rhys Blakely, "Thousands die in Tamil 'welfare village'", *The Times*, 10 July 2009.

16. Philippe Bolopion, "L'ONU a caché l'ampleur des massacres au Sri Lanka" [*The UN hid the scope of massacres in Sri Lanka*], Le Monde, 29 May 2009.

17. Jeremy Page, "British aid for war refugees may be used to fund 'concentration camps'", *The Times*, 28 Apr. 2009.

18. "Sri Lanka, stop!", *Le Monde*, editorial, 10 Sept. 2009.

19. "Sri Lanka: ICRC reiterates concern for civilians cut off by the fighting", 4 Mar. 2009, http://www.icrc.org/eng/resources/documents/interview/sri-lanka-interview-040309.htm.

20. Office of the Regional Director of Health Services, Vavuniya, "To MSF-Holland Project Coordinator. Request for Medical Team to Work at IDP Camps", 21 Apr. 2009.

21. Fabrice Weissman, "Welcome to the farm. MSF and the policy for interning the displaced people of Vanni", report of the visit to Menik Farm and Colombo camps (Sri Lanka), 4–14 June 2009. Paris, Fondation MSF/CRASH, July 2009.

22. In July 2009, the president stated his belief in "my theory…[that] there are no minorities in Sri Lanka, there are only those who love the country and those who don't", cf., *The Hindu*, 6 July 2009.

ETHIOPIA: A FOOL'S GAME IN OGADEN

1. Jeffrey Gettleman, "In Ethiopian Desert, Fear and Cries of Army Brutality", *The New York Times*, 18 June 2007.

2. MSF, "MSF Denied Access to Somali Region of Ethiopia despite Worsening Humanitarian Crisis", press release, 4 Sept. 2007.

3. "Ethiopia Blocking Civilian Access to Medicine in Conflict Zone, Agency Says", *Associated Press*, 4 Sept. 2007.

4. "Ethiopia: Government Denies 'Blocking' NGO", *IRIN*, Nairobi, 4 Sept. 2007.

5. "Report on the Findings from the UN Humanitarian Assessment Mission to the Somali Region, 30 Aug.–5 Sept. 2007".

6. "Letter from MSF International Office Secretary-General to Ethiopian Prime Minister and Minister of Foreign Affairs", 31 Mar. 2008.

7. MSF-Switzerland, "Ethiopia: Repeated Obstructions Lead MSF-Switzerland to Pull Out from Fiq, Somali Region of Ethiopia", press release, 10 July 2008.

8. MSF, "Access and Response in the Somali Region: Mission Impossible? The Case of MSF-Switzerland in Fiq", report, Dec. 2007–June 2008.

9. Letter from Tekeda Alemu, Ethiopian minister of foreign affairs, to the heads of mission of the Belgian, Dutch, Swiss and Spanish sections of MSF, 18 Feb. 2008.

10. Peter Gill, *Famine and Foreigners: Ethiopia since Live Aid*, Oxford: Oxford University Press, 2010.

11. "Ethiopia Slams Swiss Charity over Ogaden Pull-out", *Reuters*, 12 July 2008.

12. See infra, "Somalia: Everything is open for negotiation", pp. 77–106.

YEMEN: A LOW PROFILE

1. Patrice Chevalier, "The Yemeni Law and How to Use it Against Journalists", http://hal.archivesouvertes.fr/docs/00/36/17/00/PDF/Chevalier_The_Yemeni_Law_and_How_to_Use_it_Against_Journ_.pdf—version 1, 16 Feb. 2009.
2. Chevalier, "The Yemeni Law", http://hal.archivesouvertes.fr/docs/00/36/17/00/PDF/Chevalier_The_Yemeni_Law_and_How_to_Use_it_Against_Journ_.pdf—version 1.
3. www.nashwannews.com. See Samy Dorlian, "Yémen: observation sur le traitement médiatique de la guerre de Saada", Olfa Lamloum (ed.), *Médias et islamisme*, Beirut: Presses de l'Ifpo, 2010, Coll. Études contemporaines.
4. Yemen National Information Center, http://www.yemen-nic.info/news/detail.php?ID=23227. Cited in "All Quiet on the Northern Front?", New York: Human Rights Watch, Mar. 2010, p. 29.
5. MSF, La Mancha Agreement, Athens, 2006.
6. MSF internal report, Dec. 2009.
7. Interview with deputy director of communications, MSF-France, Jan. 2011.

2. AFGHANISTAN: REGAINING LEVERAGE

1. MSF press release, "After 24 Years of Independent Aid to the Afghan People, Doctors Without Borders Withdraws from Afghanistan Following Killings, Threats, and Insecurity", 28 July 2004.
2. Transcript of the press conference, July 2004, MSF archives.
3. Cheryl Benard, "Afghanistan Without Doctors", *The Wall Street Journal*, 12 Aug. 2004. Cheryl Benard's husband was then the US ambassador to Afghanistan.
4. Dr Rowan Gillies, "The Real Reasons MSF left Afghanistan", letter to the editor, *The Wall Street Journal*, 19 Aug. 2004.
5. Comment made by Colin Powell at a State Department press conference, Washington DC, 26 Oct. 2001.
6. For instance: MSF press release, "Médecins Sans Frontières casts doubt on military's 'humanitarian airdrops' in Afghanistan", 8 Oct. 2001; Rony Brauman, "Des mots magiques aux cruelles désillusions", *Le Monde*, Nov. 22, 2001.
7. See Jean-Hervé Bradol, "Questions gênantes à une coalition au-dessus de tout soupçon", *La Croix*, 17 Dec. 2001 and MSF-France president's Moral Report, May, 2002, MSF archives.
8. Department of State, Department of Defense, USAID, *Provincial Reconstruction Teams in Afghanistan: An Interagency Assessment*, June 2006, p. 10.
9. Fiona Terry, *Condemned to Repeat? The Paradox of Humanitarian Action*, London: Cornell University Press, 2002, pp. 71–80; Olivier Roy, "L'hu-

manitaire en Afghanistan: entre illusions, grands desseins politiques et bricolage", *CEMOTI*, No. 29, Jan.–June 2000, pp. 21–30.

10. MSF-France president's Moral Report, 1989, MSF archives.
11. Ahmed Rashid, *Descent into Chaos. How the War Against Islamic Extremism is Being Lost in Pakistan, Afghanistan and Central Asia*, London: Penguin Books, 2008.
12. Gilles Dorronsoro, *The Taliban's Winning Strategy in Afghanistan*, Washington: Carnegie Endowment for International Peace, 2009.
13. UNAMA, *Afghanistan: Annual Report on Protection of Civilians in Armed Conflict, 2008*, Kabul: United Nations, 2009.
14. ICRC news release, "Afghanistan: ICRC facilitates release of twelve South Korean hostages", 29 Aug. 2007.
15. MSF internal report, "Strategic choices for MSF in Afghanistan", Feb. 2009, MSF archives.
16. "Health Ministry, MSF ink MoUs", *Pahjwok Afghan News*, 30 June 2009.
17. "MSF to support 2 hospitals", *Pahjwok Afghan News*, 30 June 2009.
18. Memorandum of Understanding between the Ministry of Public Health, Islamic Republic of Afghanistan and Médecins Sans Frontières, 2009.
19. "Envoy laments weak US knowledge about Taliban", *Associated Press*, 7 Apr. 2009.
20. "Rising threat to aid agencies in Afghanistan", *Global Post*, 18 Sept. 2009.
21. "US troops stormed Afghan hospital, aid group says", *CNN.com*, 7 Sept. 2009.
22. MSF Afghanistan Situational Report, Oct. 2009, MSF archives.
23. Quotes from MSF internal report, "The challenges in accessing Boost hospital in Lashkargah city, Helmand province", Nov. 2010.
24. Assessment visit report, "Afghanistan: What humanitarian space and role for Médecins Sans Frontières?" Aug. 2007, MSF archives.

PAKISTAN: THE OTHER SIDE OF THE COIN

1. International Crisis Group, *Pakistan: The Worsening IDP Crisis*, Asia Briefing, Islamabad/Brussels: ICG, 16 Sept. 2010.
2. Formerly called North-West Frontier Province (NWFP).
3. IDP Summer Bagh Camp, 10 Mar. 2010.
4. Government of NWFP, 2009. Malakand comprehensive stabilisation and socioeconomic development strategy. Swat is one of the districts of the Malakand division.
5. http://www.usaid.gov/pk/downloads/impl/ILNo.MLK.01MalakandDivision.pdf
6. MSF press release, 25 July 2010.

3. SOMALIA: EVERYTHING IS OPEN TO NEGOTIATION

1. See in particular Roland Marchal, "Mogadiscio dans la guerre civile", *Les Etudes du CERI*, no. 69, Oct. 2000.
2. We have used this term in preference to "warlord". Roland Marchal covers the latter in detail, as the term primarily used by institutions and the international media to describe the Somali leaders in charge of the warring militias. For a critical analysis of the term and the consequences of its use on the shortcomings in the analysis of the situation in Somalia, see Roland Marchal, "Warlordism and terrorism: how to obscure an already confusing crisis? The case of Somalia", *International Affairs* (83), 2007.
3. The Alliance for the Restoration of Peace and Counter-Terrorism was a coalition of political-military leaders, supported by the United States. Although it has not been established whether or not it was formed at their instigation, the alliance was supported by the US in order to counter Al Qaeda's influence in Somalia. It quickly turned into a group with a focus on combating the Islamic courts. According to International Crisis Group, the CIA is believed to have provided the ARPCT with between 100,000 and 150,000 dollars a month. (http://www.guardian.co.uk/world/2006/jun/10/rorycarroll.oliverburkeman)
4. One of the leaders of Al Shabaab, Ayro was considered to be a representative of Al Qaeda in Somalia.
5. In 2008, forty-five humanitarian workers were killed in Somalia, compared with thirty-three in Afghanistan, nineteen in Sudan and thirteen were kidnapped, Stoddard A, Harmer A, DiDomenico V. "Providing aid in insecure environments: trends in violence against aid workers and the operational response" (2009 update), Apr. 2009, London: Overseas Development Institute", 2008 was deadliest year for aid workers—study", *Reuters*, 6 Apr. 2009.
6. Resolution 1916 (2010), adopted on 19 Mar. 2010.

4. GAZA STRIP: A PERILOUS TRANSITION

1. 2007 data, WHO office, Gaza.
2. "Gaza: la politique prime sur la santé?", MSF, Sept. 2008, http://www.msf.fr.
3. "The Gaza Strip: Operation Cast Lead, Dec. 27, '08 to Jan. 18, '09", Btselem http://www.btselem.org.
4. Expression used in a letter sent to MSF by the ministry in Mar. 2010.
5. Minutes of a meeting between Hamas and MSF, Nov. 2009.
6. Interview with the director of international cooperation at the Palestinian Authority's Ministry of Health, 12 Jan. 2011
7. Strategic plan, MSF-France, 2010.
8. Interviews carried out in Dec. 2010, Jan. and Feb. 2011.
9. Rony Brauman, "La flottille de la liberté: humanitaire ou politique?", 4 June 2010 http://www.msf-crash.org.

10. Interview carried out in Tel-Aviv, 16 Jan. 2011.
11. See "Doctors without borders gave terrorist entry pass to Israel", 17 May 2007, www.israelnationalnews.com.
12. The only crossing point for pedestrians separating Israel and the Gaza Strip.
13. AIDA, "Unprecedented denial of humanitarian access to Gaza must not continue say International Agencies", www.kvinnatillkvinna.se.
14. "Palestinian Chronicles: Trapped by War", report, supplement to *Messages*, MSF newsletter, July 2002, p. 63.
15. OCHA. Special focus—Occupied Palestinian Territories, Dec. 2007.
16. Arielle Azoulay, Adi Ophir, "The ruling apparatus of control in the Occupied Territories", symposium proceedings, Jerusalem: Van Leer Institute, Apr. 2004.
17. "As the Hamas team laughs", *Haaretz*, 19 Feb. 2006.
18. "Palestinian Chronicles", *Messages*.
19. Minutes of the Board of Directors meeting, 27 Apr. 2001.
20. Minutes of the Board of Directors meeting, 26 Apr. 2002.
21. Internal paper, 2007.

5. MYANMAR: "GOLFING WITH THE GENERALS"

1. The author would like to thank Richard Horsey for his comments on an earlier draft.
2. "Prevented from working, the French Section of MSF leaves Myanmar (Burma)", Médecins Sans Frontières press release, Paris, 30 Mar. 2006.
3. In 2008, MSF-H was treating 10,000 HIV-seropositive patients and MSF-CH 1,000 with antiretroviral therapy compared with 4,000 for the government and other aid agencies combined. See "A Preventable Fate: The failure of ART scale-up in Myanmar", Amsterdam: MSF, Nov. 2008.
4. "MSF Policy for the Near Future", Amsterdam: internal document, undated (but from content, circa 1993).
5. See, for example, "The Rohingyas: forcibly repatriated to Burma", MSF-Paris, 22 Sept. 1994.
6. "Situation report, Feb.–16 Mar. 1992", Yangon, MSF-Holland.
7. "Urban Displaced Program Shwepyithar and Hlaingthayar Townships, Yangon Division, Burma (Myanmar), Jan. 1992–July 1995", MSF-Holland, 1996, p. 6.
8. "Burma (Myanmar): Evaluation of the MSF-Holland Programs", Amsterdam, 1998, p. 24.
9. "Urban Displaced Program" at note 4, p. 19.
10. "Background of MSF-H Rakhine State Project, Myanmar, 1994–1999", MSF-Holland, Maungdaw, May 1999, p. 12.
11. The study was published in an international journal as F.M. Smithuis, F. Monti, M. Grundi, A. Zaw Oo, T.T. Kyaw, O. Phe and N.J. White, *In vivo*

sensitivity of *Plasmodium falciparum* to chloroquine, sulphadoxine-pyrimethamine, and mefloquine in Rakhine State, Western Myanmar, *Transactions of the Royal Society of Tropical Medicine and Hygiene* 91 (1997), pp. 468–472.

12. "Burma Trip Report, 26 Nov.–5 Dec., 2002" (Draft).

13. E-mail correspondence between Patrick Wieland and Jean-Clément Cabrol, 31 Aug. 2007, p. 2.

14. "Activity Report 2002, Objectives 2003", MSF-France, Paris, 2002, p. 2.

15. "Myanmar Project Overview 2005", MSF-France, 2004, p. 5.

16. MSF-CH HoM (Nov. 2005–Feb. 2008) "End of Mission report", Yangon, 12 Feb. 2008, p. 22.

17. Report of Myanmar Visit June 2006, Geneva, 2006, p. 11.

18. Interview with Asis Das, former medical coordinator for MSF-France (2005 to 2006) and AZG (2007 and 2009).

19. "Why the French section of MSF has ended its activities in Myanmar", interview with the programme manager, 30 Mar. 2006, http://msf.org/msf/articles/2006/03/why-the-french-section-of-msf-has-ended-its-activities-in-myanmar.cfm (last consulted 26 Jan. 2011).

20. Cf. infra, Fabrice Weissman, "Silence heals…", pp. 177–97.

21. "A Preventable Fate: The failure of ART scale-up in Myanmar", cf. note 2.

22. Richard Horsey, *Ending Forced Labour in Myanmar: Engaging a Pariah Regime*, London: Routledge, 2011.

23. "Statement of the United Nations Country Team in Myanmar on the Occasion of UN Day", Office of the Resident and Humanitarian Coordinator, Yangon, 24 Oct. 20007.

24. "Myanmar: ICRC denounces major and repeated violations of international humanitarian law", ICRC press release no. 07/82, Yangon/Geneva, 29 June 2007.

25. Violet Cho, "International Aid Groups Ask Junta to Eliminate Barriers", *Burma News Network*, 20 Oct. 2007. No MSF section signed this joint statement.

26. MSF-CH HoM (Nov. 2005–Feb. 2008) "End of Mission report", footnote 2, p. 4.

27. "Field Visit Report", Geneva: MSF Switzerland, Oct. 2007.

28. "MSF in Myanmar: Doubt and Certainties", Geneva: MSF International Office, Sept. 2008, p. 18.

29. "Les conditions de vie des Birmans ne sont pas aussi catastrophiques qu'au Darfour", Interview conducted by Christelle Magnout, TV5 Monde, Birmanie—l'humanitaire toléré, http://www.tv5.org/cms/chaine-francophone/info/Les-dossiers-de-la-redaction/birmanie-aung-san-suu-kyi-aout-2009/p-3964-Birmanie-L-humanitaire-tolere.htm (last accessed 20 Dec. 2010).

30. *CNN* newsroom transcripts, 7 Oct. 2007, http://archives.cnn.com/TRANSCRIPTS/0710/07/cnr.03.html (last accessed 10 Feb. 2011).

31. Translated from French, La section française de MSF met un terme à ses activités en Birmanie", interview with the programme manager, 30 Mar. 2006.

6. NIGERIA: PUBLIC (HEALTH) RELATIONS

1. The author of this chapter was head of mission in Nigeria in 2006.
2. Nigeria is divided into six politico-administrative zones called geopolitical zones: South South; South East; South West; North Central; North West; North East. This chapter focuses on the states of Kano and Katsina, both of which are part of the North West zone.
3. MSF-France Board of Directors, 22 Dec. 1995.
4. International medical symposium: "Operational responses to Epidemics in Developing Countries", Epicentre, MSF Foundation, organised on 25 Oct. 1996 at the Lariboisière Faculty of Medicine.
5. "Fighting disease; fostering development", WHO Annual Report, 1996.
6. *Impact Médecin Hebdo*, no. 339—25 Oct. 1996.
7. Moral report by president of MSF-F, 1998.
8. Guy Nicolas, "Géopolitique et religions au Nigeria", *Hérodote*, Paris: La Découverte, 2002, pp. 81–122.
9. Unicef fact sheet, 2006.
10. "Why Dr Dere Awosika should go", *Daily Trust*, Nov. 2005.
11. National Immunization Coverage Survey (NICS), 2003. Results of a survey of immunisation coverage among children aged twelve to twenty-three months.
12. FBA Health System Analysts, 2005, "The state of routine immunisation services in Nigeria and reasons for current problems", Nigeria.
13. FBA Health System Analysts, "The state of routine immunisation services...".
14. Federal Ministry of Health's National Health Management Information System (NHMIS) unit, 2006, revised policy-programme and strategic plan of action.
15. E-mail sent to the head of mission, 2004.
16. Murray Last, "The peculiarly political problem behind Nigeria's primary health care provision", University College London, 2010.
17. Elisha P. Rennes, "The limits to health intervention", *Health Transition Review*, 7, 1997, pp. 73–107; pp. 91–4.
18. Julien Claudel, Le Niger est victime d'une contrefaçon de vaccins", *La Croix*, Sept. 1996.
19. The use of Trovan for children was never approved by the FDA (Food and Drugs Administration), and its use for adults was restricted in 1999 because of its hepatic toxicity. The drug is banned in Europe.
20. Joe Stephens, "As drug testing spreads, profits and lives hang in balance", *The Washington Post*, 17 Dec. 2000.

21. Internal MSF document, country policy paper, Nigeria, Apr. 1997.
22. Evaluation conducted in 1997 by MSF-Holland.
23. Internal report, 1999.
24. Helen Cox and Siobhan Isles, "The beauty and the beast"—*The Lancet*, 2003. Sally Hargreaves, "Time to right the wrongs: improving basic health care in Nigeria", *The Lancet*, 2002.
25. "Northern Nigerian states send aid to Niger", *Agence France-Presse (AFP)*, Jul. 23, 2005.
26. E-mail correspondence between the team in Katsina and the operational team at head office, 30 Aug. 2005.
27. MSF report "Results and orientation", Aug. 2005.
28. Extract from the final report of the Katsina mission, Jan. 2006.
29. Internal MSF report, Apr. 2008.
30. Jean-Hervé Bradol, Marc Le Pape, "Innovation?", in Jean-Hervé Bradol and Claudine Vidal (eds), *Medical innovations in humanitarian situations. The work of Médecins Sans Frontières*, Médecins Sans Frontières, 2011, pp. 3–21.
31. Internal MSF document, report on operations, May 2009.
32. Since 2009, it is gradually being replaced by a conjugate vaccine which is supposed to be more effective.
33. F. Marc LaForce, Neil Ravenscroft, Mamoudou Djingarey, Simonetta Viviani, "Epidemic meningitis due to Group A Neisseria meningitis in the African meningitis belt: A persistent problem with an imminent solution", *Vaccine, the Official Journal of the International Society for Vaccines*, B13-B19, Vol. 27, Supplement 2 Jun. 24 2009.
34. Hans Veeken, Koert Ritmeijer and Benson Hausman, "Priority during a meningitis epidemic: vaccination or treatment", WHO bulletin, 1998.
35. Matthew Ferrari et al, 2009, "Katsina State meningitis outbreak: impact of the mass vaccination campaign", report Epicentre, Mar. 2010. "Time is (still) of the essence: quantifying the impact of vaccination response in Katsina State, Nigeria 2009", internal Epicentre report 2011. To allow the comparison, we have presented the percentage of averted cases in 1996 and 2009 based on the same method of calculation (described in Robert W. Pinner & al, in "Epidemic Meningococcal Disease in Nairobi, Kenya, 1989", *The journal of Infectious Diseases 1992*, pp. 359–364.)
36. Eugénie d'Alessandro, "Meningitis: From Practitioner to Prescriber", in Bradol & Vidal (eds), *Medical innovations...*, 2011.
37. Interview, Nov. 2010.
38. Dr Michel Rey, Ligue française pour la prévention des maladies infectieuses—proceedings from MSF medical symposium, 1996.

7. INDIA: THE EXPERT AND THE MILITANT

1. Ready-to-Use Therapeutic Foods (RUTF) is the generic name given to sachets of mineral- and vitamin-rich fortified milk pastes used to rehabili-

tate the nutritional status of malnourished children. Plumpy'nut, manufactured by French firm Nutriset, is a mixture of milk, groundnut, vitamins and minerals.

2. Severe acute malnutrition occurs when reserves of fat and muscle disappear as a result of inadequate supplies of energy and micronutrients. The clinical presentation includes marasmus, severe weight loss (defined in terms of variation from the anthropometric norms) and, more rarely, kwashiorkor, characterised by the presence of oedema.

3. Médecins Sans Frontières set up the Access Campaign in 1999 to improve access to medical tools and treatments suitable for pathologies the MSF teams encounter in the field.

4. "Maternal and child undernutrition: global and regional exposures and health consequences", *The Lancet*, volume 371, issue 9608, pp. 243–260, 19 Jan. 2008.

5. "'Shame' of India in its 60th year", *Daily Mail*, Aug. 2007.

6. *Indian Paediatrics*, Vol. 43, 17 Feb. 2006.

7. National Family Health Survey (NFHS)—3, 2005 to 2006.

8. Patralekha Chatterjee. "Child malnutrition rises in India despite economic boom", *The Lancet*, 369, no. 9571, pp. 1417–18.

9. Jeremy Page, "Indian children suffer more malnutrition than in Ethiopia", *The Times*, 22 Feb. 2007.

10. The Right to Food campaign will be referred to as Right to Food in this chapter. More information at http://www.righttofoodindia.org/.

11. "India bars entry of NGOs' modified Corn-Soya Blend", *Indian Express*, Express news service, 6 Mar. 2003.

12. K.S. Jayaraman, "U.S. food aid to India still under GM cloud", *CropChoice news*, in *Nature Biotechnology*, Vol. 21, no. 4, Apr. 2003.

13. Isabelle Defourny, "Operational innovation in practice: MSF's programme against malnutrition in Maradi (2001–2007)", in *A Not-So Natural Disaster: Niger 05*, Xavier Crombé & Jean-Hervé Jézéquel (eds), London: Hurst and Company, 2009.

14. Leena Menghaney, "Winners and losers in India, a major crisis in a booming economy", MSF website, Mar. 2008.

15. Plumpy'nut is protected by several patents owned by Nutriset until 2021 in twenty-nine countries, not including India.

16. "Not Biscuits, Cooked Food in Mid-Day Meal Scheme: Minister", *Thaindian News*, 17 Mar. 2008.

17. "Media Brief. People call Upon GAIN to Leave India and Government of India to Regulate PPPs", *CNN* report, 16 Apr. 2008.

18. Arun Gupta, "Commercialising young child feeding in the globalised world: Time to call for an end!!", 2009, www.rtfn-watch.org.

19. Gupta, "Commercialising young child...", 2009.

20. Retrospective mortality, nutrition and measles vaccination coverage survey, Dharbanga district, Bihar state, India. June 2008, MSF-Spain, Epicentre.

21. Livelihoods and risk of malnutrition in Dharbanga, Bihar. MSF report, Apr. 2008.
22. Jean-Hervé Bradol, Jean-Hervé Jézéquel, "Child undernutrition: advantages and limits of a humanitarian medical approach", part of the *Cahiers du CRASH* collection, p. 18.
23. "India: MSF comienza a tratar pacientes de kala azar", [India: MSF begins treating patients with kala azar], MSF press release, Aug. 2007.
24. Bradol & Jézéquel, "Child undernutrition: advantages and limits...", pp. 39–40.
25. MSF internal visit report, MSF, Aug. 2008.
26. *Indian Paediatrics*, Volume 43, 17 Feb. 2006.
27. CIPLA is an Indian pharmaceutical laboratory specialising in the production of generic medicines and Compact a Norwegian company specialising in the production of high-energy biscuits and nutritional supplements.
28. MSF visit report, Dec. 2008.
29. "India tries new way to reach its underfed children", *Reuters*, 18 Mar. 2008.
30. NFHS-3. 2005–6.
31. Right to Food Campaign Madhya Pradesh support group, "Moribund ICDS", pp. 22–23.
32. C.K. Chandrappan, starred question, 25 Feb. 2009.
33. *Indian Paediatrics*, Vol. 47, 17 Aug. 2010.
34. *Indian Paediatrics*, 2010.

SOUTH AFRICA: MSF, AN AFRICAN NGO?

1. For a more detailed analysis, see Jean-Hervé Bradol, Élizabeth Szumilin, "AIDS: A new pandemic leading to new medical and political practise", in Jean-Hervé Bradol & Claudine Vidal (eds), *Medical innovations in humanitarian situation. The work of Médecins Sans Frontières*, Médecins Sans Frontières, 2011.
2. John Donnelly, "Prevention Urged in AIDS Fight; Natsios Says Fund Should Spend Less on HIV Treatment", *Boston Globe*, 7 June 2001.
3. Khayelitsha annual activity report 2008–2009, Médecins Sans Frontières/University of Cape Town.
4. Jean-Pierre Dozon, "De l'intolérable et du tolérable dans l'épidémie de sida. Un parallèle entre l'Occident et l'Afrique", in Didier Fassin & Patrice Bourdelais (eds), *Les constructions de l'intolérable. Études d'anthropologie et d'histoire sur les frontières de l'espace moral*, Paris: La Découverte, 2005, pp. 195–224.
5. A term derived from the negationism of the extermination of Jews during the Second World War.
6. See Kerry Cullinan & Anso Thom (eds), *The Virus, Vitamins and Vegetables: The South African Aids Mystery*, South Africa: Jacana, 2009.

7. "ANC fears 'bio warfare' in Aids drug imports", *The Star*, 31 Jan. 2002.
8. Interview with Eric Goemaere, Jan. 2011.
9. "In response to SA government's reluctance towards Brazilian ARV drugs", 6 Feb. 2002.
10. Interview with the director of operations, MSF-Belgium, Jan. 2011.
11. Evaluation report, 2007.
12. "No refuge, access denied: medical and humanitarian needs of Zimbabweans in South Africa", MSF, June 2009.
13. E-mail, Dec. 2009.

FRANCE: MANAGING THE "UNDESIRABLES"

1. See Father Joseph Wresinski's report to the French Economic and Social Council, Feb. 1987.
2. MSF-France, Board of Directors, 16 Dec. 1994.
3. Respite beds were for the homeless, not sufficiently ill to be admitted to hospital emergency services but too ill to be admitted to emergency accommodation shelters.
4. MSF-France, Board of Directors, 4 Oct. 1996.
5. Basic universal healthcare coverage (Couverture maladie universelle-CMU) provides access to state healthcare coverage to all those legally resident in France with proof of three months of uninterrupted residence, who have no other access to state healthcare coverage.
6. MSF-France, Annual Report, 2000–2001.
7. State medical aid has been available since the late nineteenth century under the name of Free Medical Aid (Aide médicale gratuite-AMG). Initially intended to provide free healthcare to the destitute, since the adoption of the CMU, it is now exclusively for undocumented immigrants.
8. MSF-France, Annual Plan, 2006.
9. MSF-France, Board of Directors, 15 Dec. 2006.
10. MSF-France, Board of Directors, 2006.
11. Interview with the head of mission, Nov. 2010.
12. Eric Besson's speech in Calais, 23 Apr. 2009. http://www.immigration.gouv.fr/spip.php?page=actus&id_rubrique=254&id_article=1568.
13. http://www.lacroix.com/illustrations/Multimedia/Actu/2009/4/8/lettreassociations.pdf
14. Didier Fassin, "Une souffrance dévoilée" in Didier Fassin, *La raison humanitaire*, Paris: Hautes Etudes—Gallimard-Seuil, Paris, 2010, p. 61.
15. See also Aurélie Windels, Eric Fassin, "Eric Besson et le délit de solidarité: La loi et la jungle", *Politis*, 20 Apr. 2009.
16. The word "suffering" occurs thirty-one times in the project's Annual Report, "Support and Healthcare Centre-Paris, 2009 Activity Report", MSF, 2009.

PART TWO: HISTORY

8. SILENCE HEALS... FROM THE COLD WAR TO THE WAR ON TERROR, MSF SPEAKS OUT: A BRIEF HISTORY

1. Anne Vallaeys, *Médecins Sans Frontières: La biographie*, Paris: Fayard, 2004, p. 236.
2. Vallaeys, *Médecins sans frontières: La biographie*, p. 248.
3. Vallaeys, *Médecins sans frontières: La biographie*, p. 321.
4. Rony Brauman, "Les liaisons dangereuses du témoignage humanitaire et des propagandes politiques", in Marc Le Pape, Johanna Siméant, and Claudine Vidal (eds), *Crises extrêmes. Face aux massacres, aux guerres civiles et aux génocides*, Paris: La Découverte, 2006, pp. 188–204.
5. Anne Vallaeys, *Médecins sans frontières: La biographie*, p. 417.
6. Ibid., 441.
7. Cf., for example, Claude Malhuret, "Report from Afghanistan", *Foreign Affairs*, Winter 1983/84 (1983), pp. 426–435.
8. Cf. Justin Vaïsse, *Histoire du néoconservatisme aux États-Unis: Le triomphe de l'idéologie*, Paris: Odile Jacob, 2008, pp. 155–58.
9. Rony Brauman, cited in Laurence Binet, *Famine and forced relocations in Ethiopia—1984–1986*, Paris: MSF International Council—CRASH/MSF Foundation, Jan. 2005, p. 64.
10. Rony Brauman, *Rapport moral*, Paris: MSF, 1987.
11. Rony Brauman, *Le tiers-mondisme en question*, Paris: Olivier Orban, 1986.
12. Médecins Sans Frontières, "Candidature au prix des Droits de l'homme du Conseil de l'Europe", 20 Dec. 1988.
13. Médecins Sans Frontières, "Candidature au prix des Droits...", 1988.
14. François Jean, "Populations en danger: les propositions de MSF", *Messages*, no. 5, Dec. 1992.
15. Jacques de Milliano, "Foreword", in François Jean (ed.), *Life, Death and Aid. The Médecins Sans Frontières Report on World Crisis Intervention*, London: Routledge, 1993, p. viii.
16. François Jean, "Introduction", in François Jean (ed.), *Life, Death and Aid...*, pp. 7–8.
17. Guy Hermet, "Les États souverains au défi des droits de l'Homme", in François Jean (ed.), *Face aux crises...*, p. 191.
18. Cf. Xavier Bougarel, *Bosnie, anatomie d'un conflit*, Paris: La Découverte, 1996, pp. 11–12.
19. Anne Vallaeys, *Médecins sans frontières: La biographie*, p. 686.
20. Cf. for instance, Rony Brauman, "Introduction", in François Jean (ed.), *Populations in Danger*, London: John Libbey, 1992, p. 5.
21. Anne Vallaeys, *Médecins sans frontières: La biographie*, p. 666.
22. Françoise Bouchet-Saulnier, "Peacekeeping Operations Above Humanitarian Law", in François Jean (ed.), *Life, Death and Aid...*, pp. 128, 130.

23. See, for example, Bougarel, *Bosnie, anatomie d'un conflict*, p. 17.

24. Rony Brauman, *Le crime humanitaire. Somalie*, Paris: Arléa, 1993, p. 31.

25. Cf. for instance, Guy Hermet, "Rwanda: l'outrage humanitaire", in François Jean (ed.), *Populations en danger 1995. Rapport annuel sur les crises majeures*, Paris: La Découverte, 1995, pp. 94–95.

26. Appeal by MSF-France published in *Le Monde*, 18 June 1994.

27. *Libération*, 15 Nov. 1994.

28. Philippe Biberson, rapport moral 1996/1997, MSF, Paris.

29. François Jean, "Introduction", in François Jean (ed.), *Life, Death and Aid...*, p. 7.

30. These UN operations took place, in particular, in the Democratic Republic of Congo (1999), Liberia (2003), Haiti (2004), Côte d'Ivoire (2004), Burundi (2004), and Sudan (2005).

31. "We the Peoples: the Role of the United Nations in the 21st Century", Millennium Report of the Secretary-General of the United Nations, 2000. [http://www.un.org/millennium/sg/report/].

32. United Nations, press release, New York, 1 July 2002.

33. Michael Barry, "L'humanitaire n'est jamais neutre", *Libération*, 6 Nov. 2001.

34. Jean-Hervé Bradol, "Introduction", in Fabrice Weissman (ed.), *In the Shadow of 'Just Wars': Violence, Politics, and Humanitarian Action*, London: Hurst & Company, 2004, p. 12.

35. Fabrice Weissman (ed.), *In the Shadow of 'Just Wars'*, p. 18.

36. Judith Soussan, *MSF and Protection: Pending or Closed? Discourses and practice surrounding the 'protection of civilians'*, Paris: CRASH/Foundation MSF, July 2008.

37. Kate Mackintosh, "The development of the International Criminal Court: some implications for humanitarian action", *Humanitarian Exchange Magazine*, Issue 32, Dec. 2005.

38. Jean-Hervé Bradol, "Une commission d'enquête sur Srebrenica!", *Le Monde*, 13 July 2000.

39. Françoise Bouchet-Saulnier, "Les actions militaro-humanitaires: vrais problèmes et faux débats", Coëtquidan colloquium on international humanitarian law, organised by the French Ministry of Defence, May 2001.

40. Eric Dachy, "Justice and Humanitarian action: A Conflict of Interest", in Fabrice Weissman (ed.), *In the Shadow of 'Just Wars'...*, p. 318.

41. International Coalition for the ICC, "The role of NGOs", http://www.icc-now.org/?mod=roleofngos, consulted on 2 Apr. 2009.

42. See, for example, Fabrice Weissman, "Humanitarian aid and the International Criminal Court: Grounds for divorce", *Making Sense of Sudan*, http://blogs.ssrrc.org, July 2009.

43. Fabrice Weissman, "Not In Our Name: Why Médecins Sans Frontières Does Not Support the 'Responsibility to Protect'", 2010, *Criminal Justice Ethics*, 29: 2, pp. 194–207.

44. Cf. UN press release, 7 Apr. 2004.
45. Cf. Fabrice Weissman, "'Urgence Darfour'. Les artifices d'une rhétorique néoconservatrice", in Olfa Lamloun (ed.), *Médias et islamisme*, Beirut: Presses de l'IFPO, 2010, pp. 113–132.
46. AFP, 19 Sept. 2004.
47. AFP, 29 Oct. 2004.
48. Jean-Hervé Bradol, *Le Quotidien du Médecin*, 19 July 2004.
49. "Sudan expels 10 aid NGOs and dissolves 2 local groups", *Sudan Tribune*, 5 Mar. 2009.
50. Jean-Hervé Bradol, "The Sacrificial International Order and Humanitarian Action", in Fabrice Weissman (ed.), *In the Shadow of 'Just Wars'...*, pp. 1–22.

9. CARING FOR HEALTH

1. MSF's first charter, drafted in 1971, MSF Board of Directors archives, Paris.
2. MSF charter, amended in 1992,www.msf.fr.
3. Charles-Edward Amory Winslow, The untilled fields of public health", *Science*, 1920, 51: 23–33.
4. Charles-Edward Amory Winslow, "The untilled fields of public health", *Science*, 1920, 51: 23–33, quoted in Karen Buhler-Wilkerson, "Public health nursing: in sickness or in health?", *American Journal of Public Health*, 1985, 75: 1155–1161.
5. The World Health Organization is governed by 193 State parties, which meet once a year at the World Health Assembly (WHA).
6. Anne Vallaeys, *Médecins Sans Frontières. La biographie*, Paris: Fayard, 2004.
7. Minutes from the peer group management meeting on 31 Jan. 1973, MSF, Paris.
8. www.trumanlibrary.org/calendar/viewpapers.php?pid=1030.
9. In 1974, the United Nations General Assembly adopted a declaration concerning the establishment of a New International Economic Order (NIEO), one of whose objectives was to address development issues related to the cost of raw materials.
10. Rony Brauman (ed.), *Le Tiers-Mondisme en question*, Paris: Olivier Orban, 1986.
11. Alain Destexhe (ed.), *Santé, médicaments et développement. Les soins primaires à l'épreuve des faits*, Paris: Fondation Liberté Sans Frontières publications, 1987, p. 12.
12. "Introduction", in François Jean (ed.), *Populations in Danger*, London: John Libbey, 1992.
13. Claudine Vidal, Jacques Pinel, "'Satellites': A Strategy Underlying Different Medical Practices", Jean-Hervé Bradol & Claudine Vidal (eds), *Med-*

ical innovations in humanitarian situations, The work of Médecins Sans Frontières, Médecins Sans Frontières, 2011, pp. 22–39.

14. Approximately 200,000 people.

15. Vincent Brown, "Impact des grands slogans des Nations unies sur les programmes d'assistance technique de Médecins Sans Frontières", MSF internal report, Paris, 1991, p. 17.

16. Eric Goemaere, "Une ONG au ministère", in Rony Brauman (ed.), *Utopies sanitaires*, Paris: Le Pommier, 2000.

17. Destexhe (ed.), *Santé, médicaments et développement*, p. 10.

18. XVIIth general assembly of Médecins Sans Frontières, president's report by Dr Rony Brauman, op. cit, p. 5.

19. Philippe Biberson (president of MSF-France from 1994 to 2000), "Le désert sanitaire", in Rony Brauman (ed.), *Utopies sanitaires*, op. cit., pp. 93, 95, 96.

20. "Introduction", in François Jean (ed.), *Populations in Danger*, 1992, op. cit., pp. 3–9.

21. Jeanm "Refugees and displaced persons...", pp. 121–6.

22. Pellagra is a disease caused by malnutrition (vitamin PP or trytophane deficiency), which in the most serious cases can lead to dementia and death.

23. Alain Moren, Dominique Lemoult, "Pellagra cases in Mozambican refugees", *The Lancet*, 1990; 335, pp. 1403–4.

24. "12 ans auprès des enfants en situation difficile à Tananarive. Les raisons de la fermeture et le bilan du programme", MSF, Paris, 2005, www.msf.fr.

25. Joshua Lederberg, Robert E. Shope and Stanley C. Oaks, Jr., *editors*, *Emerging Infections: Microbial Threats to Health in the United States*, Committee on Emerging Microbial Threats to Health, Division of Health Sciences Policy, Division of International Health, Institute of Medicine, National Academy Press, Washington D.C., 1992.

26. "The Global Infectious Disease Threat and Its Implications for the United States", John C. Gannon, Chairman, National Intelligence Council, CIA, NIE 99–17D, Jan. 2000.

27. International medical symposium, MSF internal document, Paris, 20 Oct. 1996.

28. After the symposium, this issue became the subject of a publication: Dr Patrice Trouiller, Piero Olliaro, Els Torreele, James Orbinski, Richard Laing, Nathan Ford, "Drug development for neglected diseases: a deficient market and a public-health policy failure", *The Lancet*, Volume 359, Issue 9324, pp. 2188–94, 22 June 2002.

29. Marc Le Pape, Isabelle Defourny, "Controversy as a policy", in Jean-Hervé Bradol and Claudine Vidal (eds), *Medical innovations in Humanitarian situations*, Médecins Sans Frontières, 2011.

30. In 1998, a coalition of forty or so pharmaceutical laboratories took the South African government to court in an attempt to prevent it from applying a law passed in 1997 in favour of the production of generic medicines. The suit was dropped in 2001 after the waging of an opinion campaign supported by MSF.

31. Paul Blustein, "Getting out in front on trade: New U.S. representative adds 'values' to his globalization plan", *The Washington Post*, 13 Mar. 2001.

32. Cf. supra "The expert and the militant", pp. 147–60.

33. See, for example, Joan Tronto, *Moral Boundaries: A Political Argument for an Ethic of Care*, New York: Routledge, 1993.

10. NATURAL DISASTERS: "DO SOMETHING!"

1. Paul S. Auerbach et al., "Civil-military Collaboration in the Initial Medical Response to the Earthquake in Haiti", *The New England Journal of Medicine*, Feb. 2010.

2. Notably led by Prof Anthony Redmond and Dr Simon Mardel, HCRI, University of Manchester.

3. Lieutenant General Ahmed Nadeem and Andrew Mc Leod, "Non-interfering coordination: the key to Pakistan's successful relief effort", *Liaison Online* 4, no. 1 (2008)

4. Grégory Quénet, "Catastrophe naturelle", in Yves Dupont (ed.), *Dictionnaire des risques*, Paris: Armand Colin, 2007.

5. To be more precise, MSF-France's activities were suspended in Niger in 2008 on the orders of the head of state two years after the public controversies, but directly related to them.

6. Respectively, François Jean, (ed.), MSF, 1986; Xavier Crombé & Jean-Hervé Jézéquel (eds), London: Hurst and Co., 2009.

7. "Final Report of the Independent Panel of Experts on the Cholera Outbreak in Haiti", May 2011.

8. "WHO warns up to five million people without access to basic health services", 30 Dec. 2004.

9. C. de Ville de Goyet, Stop Propagating Disaster Myths, *The Lancet*, 2000, 356: 762–4, Nathalie Floret et al., "Negligible Risk for Epidemics after Geophysical Disasters", *Emerging Infectious Diseases*, www.cdc.gov/eid, Vol. 12, 4 Apr. 2006.

10. Gareth Evans, "Facing up to our responsibilities, *The Guardian*, 12 May 2008

11. *The New York Times*, 14 May 2008.

12. Bernard Kouchner, "Birmanie: morale de l'extrême urgence", *Le Monde*, 19 May 2008.

13. John D. Kraemer, Dhrubajyoti Bhattacharya, Lawrence O. Gostin, "Blocking humanitarian assistance: a crime against humanity?", *The Lancet*, Vol. 372, 4 Oct. 2008.

14. Frédérique Leichter-Flack, "Sauver ou laisser mourir", http://www.laviedesidees.fr.
15. http://www.theworld.org/2010/02/doctors-face-ethical-decisions-in-haiti/.
16. Sandrine Revet, "Anthropologie d'une catastrophe, Les coulées de boue au Venezuela", *Presses Sorbonne Nouvelle*, 2007, p. 267.
17. "Death toll from the earthquake could reach 300,000, according to the president of Haiti", *Le Monde*, 22 Feb. 2010.
18. Encounters by the author in Port-au-Prince in June 2010.
19. Peter Andreas, Kelly M. Green (eds), *Sex, Drugs and Body Count, The Politics of Numbers in Global Crime and Conflict*, New York: Cornell University Press, 2010.

EPILOGUE

1. Cyril Lemieux, *Le Devoir et la Grâce*, Paris: Economica, 2009, p. 85–89.
2. Albert O. Hirschman, *Exit, Voice and Loyalty*, Cambridge, Mass.: Harvard University Press, 1970, p. 78.
3. Albert O. Hirschman, *A Propensity to Self-Subversion*, Cambridge, Mass.: Harvard University Press, 1995, p. 12–14.
4. Albert O. Hirschman, *The Rhetoric of Reaction*, Cambridge, Mass., and London, England: The Belknap Press of Harvard University Press, 1991, p. 164.
5. MSF-Switzerland, Addis Ababa/Geneva, 10 July 2008.
6. MSF, "Commission Dasem: dernière chance pour les étrangers malades en France?" Paris, 3 May 3 2011, http://www.msf.fr/presse/communiques/commission-dasem-derniere-chance-etrangers-malades-en-france.
7. For example, Ethiopia in 1985, Zaire in May 1997 (regarding the tracking down of Rwandan refugees), North Korea in Sept. 1998, etc.
8. Marie-Pierre Allié, "Après la TB, le VIH, le diabète, demain le cancer?", *Borderline*, no. 1, MSF, Paris, Mar. 2011.
9. "Severe child malnutrition hits Nigeria's far north", *Reuters*, 26 July 2005. http://nm.onlinenigeria.com/templates/?a=3990&z=12.
10. Carlo Ginzburg, *Rapports de force*, Paris: Hautes Études, Gallimard, Seuil, 2003, p. 112. For a detailed analysis of the policy undertaken in Niger in response to the nutritional crisis, see Xavier Crombé, Jean-Hervé Jézéquel, *A Not-so Natural Disaster: Niger 05*, London: Hurst & Co., 2009.
11. Hirschman, *The Rhetoric of Reaction*, p. 45.
12. MSF, internal publication, Mar.–Apr. 2009.
13. The term "national staff" refers to MSF employees from the country in which the intervention takes place.
14. Fabrice Weissman, "Welcome to the Farm: MSF and the confinement of IDPs in the Vanni", Paris, July 2009.

15. Hirschman, *The Rhetoric of Reaction*, p. 244. Hirschman attributes the argument of imminent danger to the "repertoire of progressive rhetoric" that is, "[progressives] typically perceive the dangers of *inaction*, rather than those of action". (p. 243).

16. For a description of the circumstances in which the argument of imminent danger was used in Niger, see Marc Le Pape, Isabelle Defourny, "Controversy as a Policy", Jean-Hervé Bradol, Claudine Vidal, *Medical Innovations in Humanitarian Situations: the Work of Médecins Sans Frontières*, Médecins Sans Frontières, 2009.

17. Regarding confrontations related to the introduction of artemisin derivatives and antiretrovirals, see Suna Balkan, Jean-François Corty, "Malaria, Introducing ACT from Asia to Africa", and Jean-Hervé Bradol, Elizabeth Szumilin "Aids, a New Pandemic Leading to New Medical and Political Practices", Jean-Hervé Bradol, Claudine Vidal, ibid.

18. See Françoise Bouchet-Saulnier, *The Practical Guide to Humanitarian Law*, Maryland: Rowan & Littlefield, 2007.

19. The choice among realism, confrontation and abstention creates tensions within the MSF movement and its sections; knowledge of/familiarity with these internal debates and conflicts would require specific investigations, which is why they are rarely referred to in this study.

20. Michel Feher, "Les gouvernés en politique, *Vacarme*, 34, winter 2006. www.vacarme.org.

21. MSF, La Mancha agreement, 25 June 2006. This agreement is a "reference document" that describes those aspects of actions that are "both medical and humanitarian" on which all MSF sections agree. www.msf.fr.

22. MSF, La Mancha agreement, 2006.

AFTERWORD

1. Though obviously much distinguishes the two cases, one element of France's failure to retain control of Algeria during roughly the same period was its over-emphasis on the military and intelligence aspects of the fight—as set out by Col. Trinquier and other French officers of the period—and its neglect of the "hearts and minds" element.

2. The use of MSF's reports about Darfur by Luis Moreno Ocampo, the chief prosecutor of the International Criminal Court, in preparing his indictment against President Al Bashir of Sudan, also contributed to the association's increasing public reticence, since it had the effect of making MSF a "witness" against Al Bashir, which was the last thing that these reports had been meant to achieve.

INDEX

Abacha, Sani: regime of, 135
Abdullah, Fareed: provincial director of AIDS programme in Cape Province, 165
Achmat, Zackie: 165; founder of TAC, 164
Action Contre la Faim (ACF): 20; employees executed by government forces (2006), 18–19; members of, 179
Action Internationale Contre la Faim: founding of (1979), 202
Adventist Development and Relief Agency (ADRA): 91
Afghanistan: 3, 8, 51, 56, 182, 254; Abu-Ghraib prison, 191, 194; Badghis province, 54, 56; Ghazni, 54; government of, 58; Haqqani Network, 61, 64; Helmand province, 50, 58, 60–1, 63; Islamic Emirates of Afghanistan (IEA), 60–2, 64–5, 241; Kabul, 49–50, 53, 55, 57–8, 60–2, 255; Kandahar, 54; Kunduz, 64; Ministry of Public Health (MOPH), 52–3, 58–9; MSF members killed in, 1, 49, 191, 241; Nawzad, 63; Operation Enduring Freedom, 9–10, 50–1, 64, 189; Qala-e-Jangi, 52; Soviet Invasion of (1979–89),

54, 180, 202–3; Uruzgan province, 54
African National Congress (ANC): 166; criticisms of, 164
African Union: 39; Missions in Somalia (AMISOM), 79, 87, 92
Ahmed, Abdullahi Yusuf: administration of, 84
Ahmed, Sheikh Sharif Sheikh: President of Somalia, 88
Aids Law Project: role in creation of 'Declaration concerning the resolution of the refugee crisis', 168
Al Houthi, Hussein: supporters of, 41–2, 45
Al Jazeera: coverage of Saada War, 42, 44
Al Qaeda: 91
Al Rasheed Trust: activity of, 223
Algeria: government of, 191
All India Institute of Medical Sciences: 158
Allié, Marie-Pierre: president of MSF-France, 242
Alma-Alta Conference (1978): impact of, 131, 205–6; universal access to primary healthcare, 201
Angola: 180
Annan, Kofi: 194; UN Secretary-General, 190

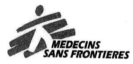
MÉDECINS SANS FRONTIERES

MSF is a movement comprised of nineteen sections based in Germany, Australia, Austria, Belgium, Canada, Denmark, Spain, the United States, France, Greece, Holland, Hong-Kong, Italy, Japan, Luxemburg, Norway, the United Kingdom, Sweden and Switzerland. Each section has its own associative structure answering to a Board of Directors elected by members during an Annual General Assembly. There are also five operational centres in France, Belgium, Holland, Switzerland and Spain. Each section defines, in keeping with MSF's charter and a series of agreements ratified by all the sections, its own intervention policies.

In 2010, MSF's resources amounted to 943 million euros, of which 90% was from private, non-governmental funding. Operational expenditure amounted to 634 million euros. The largest projects, in terms of cost, were in Haiti, the Democratic Republic of Congo, Sudan, Niger and Pakistan. Over half of MSF's programmes were conducted in situations of armed conflict or internal instability, the other half were in stable settings. MSF carried out 7.3 million out-patient consultations, cared for 360,000 hospitalised patients, treated 370,000 children suffering from malnutrition, 174,000 patients with cholera and nearly 40,000 war wounded. The organisation also provided antiretroviral treatment to 180,000 AIDS patients.

These projects were carried out by over 25,000 staff—doctors, nurses, logisticians, administrators, epidemiologists, laboratory technicians etc.—most of whom work in their own country.

For more information on Médecins Sans Frontières: www.msf.org

MEDECINS SANS FRONTIERES' CHARTER

Médecins Sans Frontières (MSF) is a private international association. The association is made up mainly of doctors and health sector workers and is also open to all other professions which might help in achieving its aims. All of its members agree to honour the following principles:

Médecins Sans Frontières provides assistance to populations in distress, to victims of natural or man-made disasters and to victims of armed conflict. They do so irrespective of race, religion, creed or political convictions.

Médecins Sans Frontières observes neutrality and impartiality in the name of universal medical ethics and the right to humanitarian assistance and claims full and unhindered freedom in the exercise of its functions.

Members undertake to respect their professional code of ethics and to maintain complete independence from all political, economic or religious powers.

As volunteers, members understand the risks and dangers of the missions they carry out and make no claim for themselves or their assigns for any form of compensation other than that which the association might be able to afford them.